C000265061

GET LEAN AND STRONG

Your complete guide to building the perfect body

By Neil Cooper

GET LEAN AND STRONG ISBN 978-1-9998728-5-4

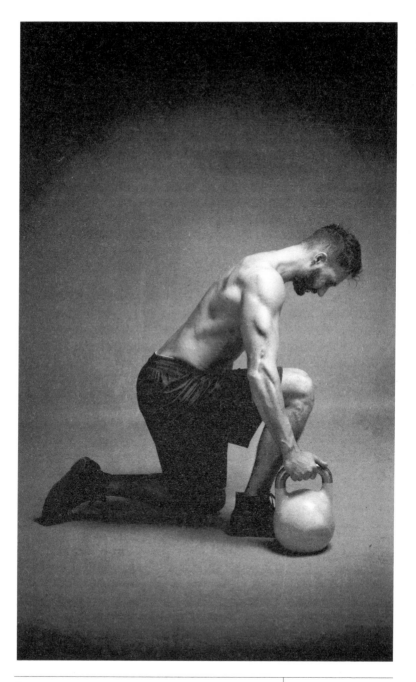

Contents

Let's get to work

Welcome to your guide to getting results

Welcome to *Get Lean And Strong, Your Complete Guide To Building The Perfect Body*. Inside this guide we've given you the essential training and nutrition information you need to reduce body fat, increase strength and add lean muscle mass. It's an important book because, frankly, there's so much poor information out there. That's one of the reasons why people are so confused about the best approach to use when they want to make a positive difference to how they look and feel.

One of the problems regarding poor fitness information is the fact that people will try to sell you the "new craze" or the "quirky class" as a way of making a name for themselves and adding to their bank balance. In reality, it's the tried-and-tested fundamentals that you need to focus on if you want to make a real change. So ignore the fads, sidestep the gimmicks and concentrate on the good stuff.

A new chapter in your training career

The book starts with a chapter that addresses and dispels some common fat loss and muscle building myths, while also giving you a grounding in the approach you need to take if you want to have success in those two areas.

The second chapter focuses on nutrition, which is a huge subject and could easily fill ten 500-page volumes. The trick, however, is to concentrate first on the stuff that really matters - the stuff that will have the biggest effect with the least amount of effort. That's always the way we think you should approach things. Devote your attention to the fundamentals and then, once you master those, you can start to add detail and make things more complicated. But if you rush in from the start with a complex approach the chances are you're going to be overwhelmed, or you'll misinterpret and misuse information and you won't get the result you want. It's much better to start with some easy wins, build the success habit and refine your approach over time. That does require a little discipline and patience at first but, trust us, you'll be well rewarded in the long run.

The next chapter outlines the key resistance training exercises that we suggest you focus on if you want to lose fat and add muscle. We detail the compound, isolation and abdominal moves that should form the basis of your training plans. Now, this is by no means an exhaustive list of exercises

that are worth doing. But unless you're already an advanced lifter in great
shape, you don't need access to an exhaustive list. You need to master
the basics, excel at the basics and then introduce new moves once you've
exhausted the benefits of the ones in this book.

The final chapter is on training theory. This will give you the information
and understanding you need to create your own training plans. We look at
how to select the right training split for your goals, how to manipulate key
workout variables and how to introduce advanced lifting protocols into your
training to ensure that your progress never stalls. It gives you the tools you
need to take your training destiny into your own hands and get great results
for years to come.

Mind and muscle

One thing we'd like to mention before you start the book is mindset. It's a
huge subject in itself but, fundamentally, when it comes to training, you're
aiming to develop your mindset as much as your muscles. That's because
as you get fitter, gains get harder to come by. Beginners will usually see
rapid improvements because they have huge potential to exploit. But as you
improve, those gains are likely to slow and that's when you need the mental
toughness to keep pushing on.

The other thing we want to highlight is that training is fairly meritocratic.
You get out what you put in. If you coast through your sessions and don't
make much of an effort then, guess what? You're not going to see great
results. But if you apply yourself consistently over time and give every rep
everything you've got then you'll be blown away by what you can achieve.
The results are there for the taking, you just need to train intelligently and
do the work.

Part 1
Introduction

The secret to burning fat and building muscle

You probably didn't think you were going to get the secret to both burning fat and building muscle quite so early in the book. But here it is: the secret to success lies in doing the training and nutrition basics consistently over time. With diet, that means eating a variety of fresh food in line with your energy intake needs. And for training it means following a progressive resistance training plan where you manipulate key training variables in line with your goals. Of course, when you dig into the real detail for those last two sentences there's a phenomenal amount to explore. But in essence the key to progress is pretty simple: apply what has been proven to work over time and you'll see results. The rest of this book will be devoted to helping you do just that but first up we'd like to dispel a few common fat burning and muscle building myths before revealing the most important concepts that you need to focus on throughout your training journey.

BEWARE THE QUICK FIX
When it comes to training and nutrition there's something we want you to remember; if it sounds too good to be true then it probably is too good to be true. A lot of people out there want a shortcut and that's something unscrupulous individuals within the fitness industry are more than happy to exploit. That's also why there's so much misinformation about nutrition and training. So beware the quick-fix promises and instead look for advice with substance.

Fat loss myths

The truth behind common fat-burning fallacies

MYTH 1: CALORIES DON'T COUNT

You hear this one all the time; you shouldn't fixate on calories and what you eat is all that matters. Well, let me put this to you. Imagine that you only eat good quality meat and fish and fruit and vegetables and nuts and seeds and all that healthy stuff. Great, right? Well what if your total calorie intake for the day comes to about 5,000 calories and your total calorie expenditure comes to about 2,500 calories. That's less great, right? Because you're consuming more than you're using and that will, ultimately, cause you to gain weight. The real story is that you shouldn't obsess over calories but the bottom line is that calories do matter.

MYTH 2: CALORIES ARE ALL THAT COUNT

At the other end of the myth spectrum is the idea that the only thing you need to worry about is your calorie intake. If we use the energy in versus energy out concept then that sounds pretty reasonable. After all, if you consume 2,500 calories a day and you use 2,500 calories a day then you're in a good energy balance. Well, let's look at it another way. If you're getting your calories from a wide variety of fresh food, that's great. But what if your calories are coming exclusively from ice cream and doughnuts. Is that just the same? In the latter case, you'll be depriving your body of the vital minerals, vitamins and other nutrients it needs to function optimally. The take away tip: calories count, but so do other factors.

MYTH 3: CARBS MAKE YOU FAT

This idea has been around for a long time and it essentially says that if you eat carbs (including grains such as bread, pasta and rice, and different forms of sugar) then you'll gain weight. The reality is that carbs do not inherently cause you to gain weight. If you eat a diet with a balance of macronutrients (proteins, carbs and fats) and you ensure that you get the vitamins and minerals that your body needs, and you take in the calories that you need but not more than you need then you'll be fine. The myth has perhaps taken root because refined carbs can be easy to overeat, and it is the overconsumption of food that will cause you to gain weight. Our advice is to try to limit your consumption of refined carbs (such as processed sugars).

TAKEAWAY TIP: Be wary of any
nutrition advice that's extreme,
excessively restrictive or
demonises entire food groups.

MYTH 4: EATING CARBS AFTER 6PM MAKES YOU FAT

This myth says that as soon as the clock hits six o'clock in the evening then
the way your body processes carbohydrates instantly changes and causes
you to gain weight. The truth is that the *overconsumption* of carbs - or indeed
any macronutrient - causes you to gain weight. The myth may have come
from the fact that if you are cutting out a whole food group in the evening
then you are perhaps likely to consume fewer calories. So it is the calorie
consumption, rather than the content of those calories, that is affecting your
body composition. There's evidence to suggest that eating a big meal late at
night is associated with weight gain but that's not carb specific.

MYTH 5: FAT MAKES YOU FAT

By now you're probably getting a good idea about the reality behind these
myths. In this case, the idea is that consuming dietary fat will make you fat.
Again, it isn't inherently true. And again, you should be more concerned
with the overconsumption of fat. It is, however, worth pointing out that not
all fats are nutritionally equal. Some fats, such as saturated, polyunsaturated
and monounsaturated fats should all be present in your diet. It's probably
a good idea to aim for a roughly equal intake of all three. The fats that
you want to avoid are called trans fats and they are commonly found in
sweets, biscuits, pastries and cakes. There is strong evidence to suggest that
consuming large quantities of trans fats can be detrimental to your health.

MYTH 6: JOGGING IS BEST FOR FAT LOSS

If you want to lose fat then the best thing you can do is lace up a pair of
running shoes and head out for a jog. This isn't total nonsense. Jogging
can have a positive impact on your body composition because it burns
calories and is a form of exercise. But is it the most effective way to burn
fat? Probably not. Our recommendation would be to undertake a resistance
training regime that includes elements that significantly raise your heart
rate. This kind of exercise will burn just as many calories as jogging (and
maybe even more) while also helping you to add muscle mass, which is
active tissue and can increase the calories you burn throughout the day.
Resistance training also offers other benefits, such as increasing bone density.

The key to fat loss

The key concepts that get results

UNDERSTAND ENERGY BALANCE

On the previous page we looked at a couple of misleading ways that calories are used when it comes to creating a fat loss strategy. The upshot is that calories do count but they are not the only thing that matters. The sensible way to look at your fat loss plan would be to ensure that you are in a small but sustainable calorie deficit while also aiming to eat a nutrient-dense diet. So, for example, you could aim to be in a calorie deficit of about 250 calories a day. You'd do that if you consumed 2250 calories and burned 2500. If you dropped your calories to about 1500 then theoretically you'd lose fat faster but you're also likely to feel hungry and that can make you feel miserable, which is unsustainable. If your approach is unsustainable then, sooner or later, you'll ditch it. And when you ditch it you won't make any progress at all and may even go backwards. So, a smart way to do things is to find a calorie deficit that's manageable. And if you do that while also eating a variety of fresh food, then you'll hit your targets and enjoy the process.

USE RESISTANCE TRAINING

The most effective fat loss plans are ones that combine a smart and sustainable nutrition plan with a progressive resistance training plan. Yes, simple cardio exercise such as jogging can have a positive impact on your waistline, but it won't do much to improve your physique from a muscle-building point of view. A better approach would be to undertake an exercise plan that involves lifting weights. You'll want to make sure that this plan is progressive, which means it gets harder as you get fitter, to ensure that your results don't stagnate. You also want to ensure that it involves training elements that increase your heart rate so you get the bonus benefits of cardio exercise without having to complete a dedicated cardiovascular training session. Of course, if you just love running and want to include a run in your weekly training schedule, that's fine. After all, enjoying your training is important.

DON'T DO ANYTHING DRASTIC

Too often, when people want to lose fat or add muscle, they opt for an extreme approach. Take crash diets, which either drastically reduce your calorie intake or cut out large food groups. They may work temporarily, either because you'll lose water weight or because you're effectively starving yourself. But in the long run they are unsustainable and therefore they are pretty worthless. Even worse, they may even have a negative impact on your physical or mental health. We'll keep saying this again and again but the real 'secret' to fat loss is doing the basic things consistently over time. The same applies to training. Going from a relatively sedentary lifestyle to doing hours and hours of exercise a day isn't the best way to achieve a result. What your body really needs is to be challenged appropriately and then be allowed to recover so that it can rebuild your muscles and connective tissue to be bigger and stronger than before.

THINK LONG TERM

You've probably seen the magazine coverlines promising 'flat abs in 7 days'. Well, they are designed to sell magazines, not to get lasting results. And what happens with your limited-time plan has ended? Do you just revert back to the lifestyle you had before? If you do then you'll revert back to the body shape you had before. But if you make small and sustainable changes and implement them over time then you will gradually adjust your habits and your lifestyle. When you do that, you can start to enjoy your workouts and enjoy the food you're eating. As we've already said, consistency is what gets results and when you see results you'll be motivated to continue. If you keep doing what you're doing then eventually it will become second nature and you'll no longer even feel like you need to make an effort. And the less effort something takes, the easier it is to sustain. If something requires a monumental effort then that can be draining and it will have a detrimental impact on your long-term results.

Muscle-building myths

Avoid these pitfalls to make faster progress

MYTH 1: YOU SHOULD ONLY TRAIN A MUSCLE ONCE A WEEK
This muscle-building myth has probably come about as a result of misinterpreting an approach to training that's used by the bodybuilding community. The idea, for example, is that on Monday you train your chest, on Tuesday you train your back and so on. You do five or six body-part sessions a week so you train each body part once a week. The theory is that if you train only one muscle group then you can fatigue it fully, which will maximise muscle growth. It is true that to build muscle you need to properly fatigue a body part but another important hypertrophy factor is volume (the amount of work you complete). When you train a muscle group twice a week, for example, your volume increases and your results can improve.

MYTH 2: MORE IS BETTER
If we extend the theory from the last point - that training a body part two times a week is more effective, from a muscle-building point of view, than training a body part once a week - then surely training it three or four times is even more effective? Well, that's not necessarily the case because it is while you're recovering from a training session that your muscles repair and grow to become bigger and stronger. If you interrupt that recovery process before it is complete then you may be compromising your results. Also, if you train a body part before you have recovered then you may not be able to lift as much weight. The lesson is that there is a happy medium and that both too much and too little will hamper your progress.

MYTH 3: YOU SHOULD CHASE MUSCLE SORENESS
Now, if you think that the sign of a good session is waking up with severe DOMS (delayed onset muscle soreness) the next day then you're in good company. Because even some experienced lifters believe this to be the case. The fact is that there is no correlation between soreness and the effectiveness of your session. Scientists are still somewhat divided over what causes muscle soreness. You're more likely to experience it if you have had a break from training and you may also feel it more severely in some muscle groups than others. Our advice is to follow a reputable plan and to execute each session to the best of your ability without fixating on soreness.

MYTH 4: NEVER DO THE SAME WORKOUT TWICE

You've probably heard different forms of this myth. But in its purest form it is that you shouldn't do the same workout twice because you need to keep your muscles 'guessing'. As with a lot of training myths, there's a kernel of truth in there somewhere. In this case, it's a distortion of the idea that you shouldn't just do the same thing over and over again. If you do that, your body will get comfortable and your results will stall. But the idea that you can never do the same workout twice is also unhelpful. It may be the case that you need a level of consolidation in your workouts. You've learned the movement pattern of an exercise, for example, and you need to keep performing it to ensure that you take advantage of your new motor skills.

MYTH 5: ISOLATION MOVES ARE A WASTE OF TIME

You know what's really a waste of time when it comes to training? Sweeping statements. Now, it is true that isolation moves are probably more important to bodybuilders than they are to strength training athletes. But isolation moves can have a place is everyone's routine. For example, if building big biceps is your goal, then bent-over rows will help you to do that. But once your back muscles fatigue in that movement you won't be able to complete a rep. When that happens, you'll need to focus directly on the biceps muscles by doing moves such as biceps curl variations. You should also be aware that only doing isolation work isn't ideal. The best programmes are ones that contain a mix of compound and isolation work.

MYTH 6: DO 3 SETS OF 10 REPS FOR MAXIMUM MUSCLE GROWTH

There's a lot of muscle-building mileage in doing three sets of 10 reps. It's working in the hypertrophy rep range and three sets will give you decent training volume. But it's only one of the set and rep ranges at your disposal. You'll maximise your results by mixing up your set and rep ranges. You could, for example, include some lower-rep work, such as doing 5 sets of 5 reps on a big compound move at the start of your session to build strength. And you could maybe throw in a couple of 20-rep sets of an isolation move at the end of your workout to safely and properly fatigue your muscles. Sets and reps are variables that you should always be looking to manipulate.

The key to building muscle

The most important hypertrophy factors

MAKE SURE YOU EAT ENOUGH

If you want to build muscle then you need to make sure that your body has the resources it needs to lay down new muscle tissue. And that means you need to eat enough to be in an anabolic state. If you fail to eat enough then you'll be in a catabolic state, which is more conducive to losing weight than building muscle. Of course, when people are trying to build muscle it is usually because they want to 'look better' and if they want to look better then they are also likely to be fearful of adding body fat. That's why a fear of adding fat can also prevent you from adding muscle. On the other hand, if you eat too much then you are likely to add body fat. And it should also be said that the food you eat will only be used to add muscle if you're training in a way that causes damage to your muscle fibres. If you just eat a load of extra food without training then you won't add muscle, you'll add fat.

LIFT HEAVY WEIGHTS

The mistake a lot of people make when they are chasing size is to overlook the importance of strength. You do need to lift in a hypertrophy rep range if you want to add size but the more weight you can lift in that range, the better. For example, which do you think will have a bigger impact on your body composition, bench pressing 50kg for 10 reps or bench pressing 100kg for 10 reps? So while you're chasing size you should also seek to build an appreciable level of strength. One simple strategy you can use is to perform a lot of your big moves such as squats, bench presses and overhead presses using either strength (1-5) or functional hypertrophy (6-8 reps) ranges. We'd probably advise against going lower then 5 reps if hypertrophy is your aim but there's a lot of value in the 5-8 rep range if you want to get bigger. You can then use higher rep ranges for your isolation work but, as ever, it makes sense to mix things up and also do your compound lifts using conventional hypertrophy rep ranges of around 8-12 and even as high as 20 reps if you want to burn fat too.

AIM TO MAXIMISE VOLUME

In training terms, volume is the total amount of work you complete, which you calculate by multiplying the sets, reps and weight that you lift. If, for example, you perform 3 sets of 10 reps with 100kg then your volume is 3x10x100, which is 3,000kg. One of the most effective ways to maximise your muscle growth is to increase your volume. This could be done by adding reps, sets or load. It can also be done by increasing frequency (how often you train). You will, however, need to be smart with how you increase volume. It is difficult to achieve a lot of volume if you are lifting using a high percentage of your one-repetition maximum. But, equally, if the percentage of your one repetition maximum is too low then you won't stimulate a muscle-building effect. The sweet spot therefore lies not just in the middle (because you don't want to just do the same thing over and over again) but in manipulating the variables to do as much high-quality work as possible.

SEE IT AS A LONG GAME

If you want real success when it comes to training then it pays to see it as a long-term game. That's even more vital when it comes to building muscle. You see, it is possible (although not necessarily desirable) to lose a significant amount of body fat in a short space of time. It's almost impossible, on the other hand, to add a serious amount of muscle (without resorting to illegal substances) in a short period of time. It's also smart to see things as a long term lifestyle evolution rather than a quick fix. There's something about the quick-fix mentality that wants something for nothing. It suggests that you're trying to take a shortcut or look for a cheat when, in reality, there isn't a way to cheat your fitness progress. When you think short-term, you're always looking for a way out but when you adopt a long-term attitude then you can be content in the knowledge that although progress may not be immediate, it will come.

Part 2
Nutrition

How to eat for your body composition goals

A lot of people are confused about nutrition, and that's understandable. There are so many contradictory (or downright incorrect) things said about the way we eat that you'd be forgiven for being unsure about how you should approach nutrition. The truth is that the facts are often more mundane than a lot of the sensational claims you read. Those claims are often made by people who want to stand out and make a name for themselves. For them, giving you accurate information may not give them the attention they crave so they feed you misinformation.

If you want a healthy approach to nutrition then you need to do the basics well. You need to eat a variety of fresh food. You need to eat good quality protein, healthy fats and a wide variety of vegetables. We'd also advise against anything extreme or cutting out whole food groups, unless you have a diagnosed intolerance. Once you've mastered those basics you can begin to get a bit more sophisticated, but do it in the knowledge that you'll have to experiment to find out what works for you and what you can sustain. When it comes to nutrition, one size does not fit all. And what one person is able to sustain may be intolerable to someone else. So take on board the advice in this section and then begin to explore and experiment until you have found the optimal approach for you.

Basic nutrition principles

Take these ideas on board to keep your diet on track

EAT A VARIETY OF FRESH FOOD

If we had to explain our philosophy for healthy eating in the simplest possible terms, it would be this: aim to eat a wide variety of fresh food. This isn't a complete instruction on the 'perfect' way to eat but it's an incredibly effective way of communicating a substantial amount of information in a few simple words. If we begin to delve deeper into why it's useful there are a couple of things that we should pick out. We recommend eating a variety of foods because that will help to ensure that you are getting all of the macronutrients and micronutrients that your body needs. Different foods contain different nutrients so it therefore makes sense to eat a variety of them. The second element focuses on eating fresh food. What we mean by this is foods that have either not been processed before you consume or cook with them. So we're thinking about foods in their natural states, such as fruits and vegetables, nuts and seeds, cuts of meat, fish and eggs. Highly processed foods, on the other hand, such as sweets, cakes and biscuits, aren't included in our recommended foods list.

EAT AS MANY VEGETABLES AS YOU LIKE

Here's something it is pretty much impossible to do: gain weight by eating too many vegetables. So when it comes to vegetables, feel free to eat as much as you like. There are a couple of reasons why it is difficult to over-consume vegetables. They are generally low in calories, so it would be almost impossible to eat 1,000 calories of vegetables. It would be annoyingly easy, on the other hand, to eat 1,000 calories of pizza. Vegetables are also high in fibre, which helps you to feel full, so if you pile your plate with veg then you're likely to feel satisfied. Now we've established that you can't really do yourself any harm by eating veg, it's time to look at the positive stuff that you can do. Vegetables are generally very nutrient dense, which means they contain loads of nutrient bang for their calorie buck. Eating vegetables will have a positive impact on pretty much every biological function in your body and

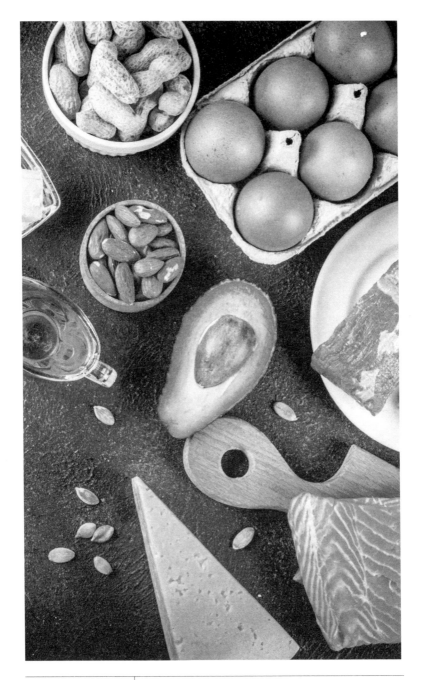

it is also likely to have a positive impact on your overall health, as well as your body composition. One quick note - when we say you can eat as much veg as you like, you should still aim to eat a variety of veg. We wouldn't, for example, recommend that you only ate carrots.

KEEP YOURSELF HYDRATED

One of the easiest things you can do to have a positive effect on your body composition is to ensure that you drink enough water. If you're dehydrated that can make you feel hungry, so drinking water will help you to avoid eating unnecessarily. Your body also needs water to carry out a host of functions, so make sure you drink throughout the day. There isn't a perfect amount of water to drink. If you're exercising regularly - and therefore sweating - then you'll want to increase your intake accordingly. A good amount to aim for is a couple of litres a day. You may also want to increase the amount you drink when it is hot, because you'll sweat more. You also lose water while you're sleeping so we recommend that you have a large glass of water soon after waking. One word of caution - some drinks can actually dehydrate you. Unsurprisingly, alcoholic drinks are the worst offenders but coffee can also dehydrate you. We also suggest that you drink water, as opposed to, say, fruit juices, because water doesn't contain calories.

THINK PROTEIN FIRST

Before we get into this properly it is worth saying that a healthy diet is one that contains a balance of proteins, carbohydrates and healthy fats. But if we had to arrange those macronutrients with body composition in mind then we'd base our meals around a high quality protein source, then add the healthy fats and finally fill in the rest of your calorie allocation with carbohydrates. There are a couple of reasons for this. If you're trying to add muscle while bulking up or preserve muscle while slimming down then it is vital that you maintain good protein intake. Healthy fats are essential for a range of important functions, such as optimising the male sex hormones which, again, is essential when you're aiming to add muscle and get lean. Carbohydrates can be thought of as useful fuel. If you don't have any fuel then you may struggle to complete your workouts with sufficient intensity. Now, there is some evidence to suggest that high fat, low carb diets, such as the Keto diet, can be effective for improving body composition but they need to be used with a high level of understanding so it's not where we'd start off with a beginner.

EVERYONE IS DIFFERENT

If anyone tells you that they have discovered the 'perfect' way to eat, they are lying to you. We can identify ways of eating that will tend to be helpful or unhelpful for different health and fitness goals but the perfect diet does not exist. One of the main reasons for this is that we are all different. For example, some people can very easily tolerate low carbohydrate diets and some people will really struggle if you reduce their carbohydrate consumption. It is also the case that some people have intolerances, such as dairy or wheat sensitivities, which should influence how they eat. Other people, however, will be easily able to tolerate those foods and therefore there is no reason for them to be avoided.

THE BEST APPROACH IS A SUSTAINABLE ONE

What's your ideal diet? It's the best diet that you're able to sustain over time. You see, if a diet has phenomenal results for four weeks but is so difficult to sustain that it causes you to fall off the wagon, binge on all of the suff you've been trying to avoid and end up in a worse place than when you started, then that phenomenal diet isn't that phenomenal, is it? That's why you should always think in terms of sustainability. Related to this is the idea that nutrition isn't just a thing that exists on paper. It's something that, because you're a human being, you have to adhere to while living your life. And in the course of your life you're going to experience different emotions that will influence how you eat. For example, if you go through a particularly challenging time, that may encourage you to eat 'comfort foods' that may be high in calories and sugar. Equally, different times of day present different challenges. It's a heck of a lot easier to stick to a 'healthy' diet on the 25th of January than it is on the 25th of December. And as a final word, what you eat on the 25th of December doesn't really matter, because you should evaluate your diet in terms of weeks or months, not days. Taking a longer view is a much healthier way, from a psychological perspective, to look at things.

Pre-workout nutrition

What to eat before training to maximise performance

MAKE IT PERSONAL

Your perfect pre-workout approach will be whatever works best for you. Some people like working out on an empty stomach and others feel like they need to eat in order to fuel their efforts. The best feedback will be how you feel during a session. If you feel terrible, something needs to change.

FOOD TIMING

The theory behind the optimal time to eat before a session says that you want to have about a 90-minute gap between a meal and a workout to give your body enough time to digest the food. The gap between eating and exercising will also be influenced by the size of your meal. Time of day will also play a part. If you have to get to the gym before work then you may not have the luxury of eating far enough in advance of your session. In that instance, an easy-to-digest snack and a coffee may be what you need. You can then have a more substantial protein-rich breakfast after your session.

POWERED BY COFFEE

If you are a coffee drinker then we'd recommend having a cup before your workout, provided you're either training in the morning or at lunchtime. If you train in the evening then the caffeine may adversely affect your sleep. Earlier in the day, however, it should provide a performance boost. There is solid research to show that caffeine can increase the focus, intensity and endurance of a session, which makes it a great pre-workout option.

PRE-WORKOUT SUPPLEMENTS

This kind of supplement is an interesting coffee alternative. Most pre-workout supplements contain caffeine, so you'll still get your kick. They also often contain other potentially useful ingredients such as Beta Alanine, which has been shown to positively impact strength endurance and muscle pump. They may also contain certain branch-chain amino acids (BCAAs), which can help to prevent muscle breakdown, particularly if you are training in a fasted state. Pre-workouts can be quite intense and produce tingling sensations (which are quite normal) so it is best to try a small dose first to see how you react and decide whether or not you like the effect.

Post-workout nutrition

Accelerate recovery with this post-workout plan

PROTEIN PRIORITY

You're probably already familiar with the idea of consuming post-workout protein. Well, it is a smart thing to do because it will help your muscle fibres repair and re-grow to become bigger and stronger. Our suggestion is to consume a generous portion of protein in your post-workout meal. You can also use a protein shake, if that's more convenient. Protein shakes aren't superior to protein-rich foods such as steaks and chicken, they're just quick and easy to consume. One thing to be aware of is the carbohydrate content of your shake. If fat loss is your primary goal then we'd advice against using a mass-gain shake, which will contain a substantial amount of carbs.

CARBOHYDRATE QUESTION

What you may be less familiar with is the idea of consuming post-workout carbs. If you're on a fat-loss push and really trying to limit calorie intake, then you may want to save the bulk of your post-workout calorie intake for protein. But if you're interested in overall performance then post-workout carbs are useful because they replace glycogen (stored energy) used during exercise and they can also facilitate muscle-protein synthesis.

NUTRIENT TIMING

This is a hotly-contested subject and recent evidence suggests that timing isn't worth fixating on, unless you're looking to extract every last ounce of benefit from the way your diet is structured. What's more important is your total daily intake. If you're an elite athlete, then timing does matter. If you're a regular gym goer, it's not the most important thing. Again, think about how sustainable it is to adhere to strict timing protocols. If it's easy enough, great. If it is causing you stress, then it's probably not worth worrying about.

DOUBLE PROTEIN HIT

If increasing muscle size is your aim, or you find it particularly hard to add muscle, then you may want to have a post-workout protein shake and then have another protein-rich meal an hour later. This isn't a necessary strategy but it is one way of ensuring that you're taking full advantage of your body's ability to synthesise protein to create bigger and stronger muscles.

Breakfast

Start the day right to eat well all day

MOST IMPORTANT MEAL?

You've probably heard that breakfast is the most important meal the day. Well, there's not much scientific evidence to support that statement. But from a psychological point of view, it can be critical because starting your day well makes it easier to continue to eat well. If you skip breakfast you also run the risk of experiencing a mid-morning energy crash and reaching for a high-sugar pick-me-up. While some people are perfectly able to skip breakfast and eat well for the rest of the day, we wouldn't recommend it as a default option.

PROTEIN MATTERS

Our suggested approach to eating means you should base all of your meals around a protein source. For breakfast, the easiest and most versatile option is to include eggs in your first meal of the day. Eggs are an excellent source of protein and healthy fats and they're quick and easy to make.

THINK AHEAD

Sometimes you might want to eat a healthy breakfast but you're running short on time. If making an omelette with vegetables, for example, is unrealistic then instead of grabbing a pastry on your way to work we advise you to think ahead. You can boil a couple of eggs the night before and eat them with a bowl of berries on the side.

HEALTHY BREAKFAST EXAMPLES

- Scrambled eggs with smoked salmon, wholemeal toast and 1/2 a grapefruit
- Ham, cheese and mushroom omelette with wholemeal toast and a banana
- Mashed avocado and fried egg on toast with a bowl of berries
- Natural yogurt with seeds and berries and a small handful of nuts
- Porridge oats with milk and a scoop of protein powder with an apple

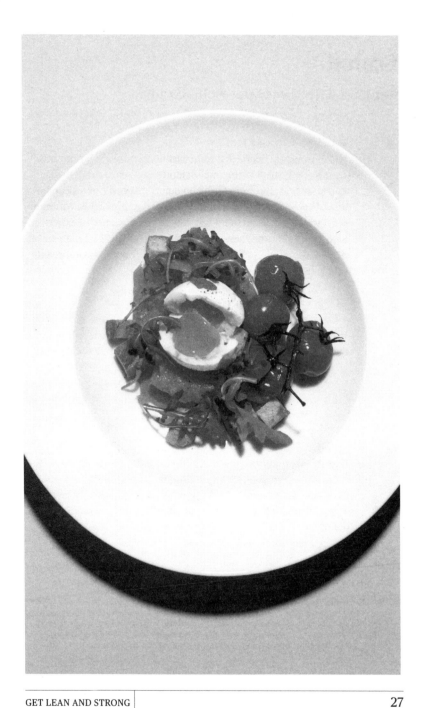

Lunch

Get lean with these speedy lunch ideas

MAKE IT YOURSELF

Making your own food is a good way of controlling the cost of your meals as well as the ingredients and portion sizes. Try to find time to make yourself a quick salad that you can take with you when you leave the house. If you're having chicken for dinner one evening, cook an extra breast and include that in a salad with sliced avocado, tomato and lettuce leaves. If you want to get fancy, make a quick dressing with clear honey, mustard and rapeseed or olive oil.

DITCH PACKAGED SANDWICHES

A lot of packaged supermarket sandwiches leave a lot to be desired from a nutrient point of view. They are often high in calories thanks to the inclusion of mayo to make up for the poor quality and taste of the meat. They're also often high in salt. So if you are going to have a sandwich, you're better off making it yourself, and using low-fat mayo or low calorie options such as mustard, to give it extra flavour.

SECRET SAUCE

A lot of salad sauces contain hidden calories, which can be unhelpful when you're trying to lose fat. Caesar and ranch dressings, for example, can contain as many calories as the rest of your salad. We're not saying that they should be completely off the menu, but you should be aware of what you're consuming so you can make informed decisions.

HEALTHY LUNCH EXAMPLES

- Chicken, avo and tomato salad with honey and mustard dressing, 1 apple
- Low-fat tuna mayonnaise sandwich on wholemeal bread and a banana
- Three-bean salad with feta cheese and a handful of grapes
- Homemade chicken Caesar salad with yogurt rather than mayonnaise
- Tuna Nicoise salad and an orange

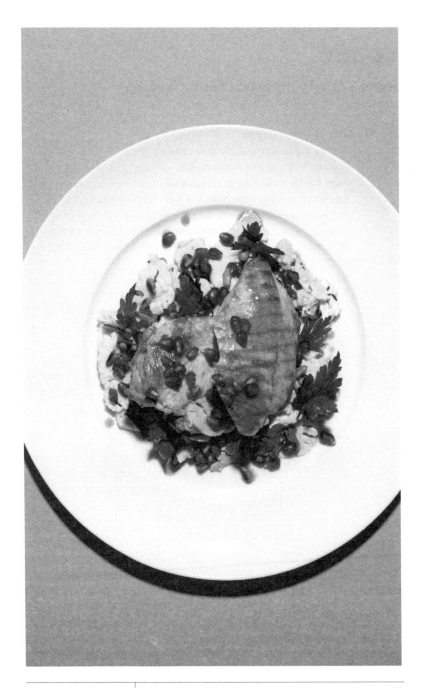

Dinner

Make a hearty dinner to finish the day strong

PROTEIN PRIORITY

Dinner is a great time to indulge in your quest for good quality protein. There are so many options, from pan-fried steaks and lamb chops to grilled chicken and fish. It allows you to keep your menus fresh and interesting. And you can have a good portion of carbs with your meal too. Don't get sucked into the myth that if you eat a potato after 6pm that you'll instantly develop a massive belly. Just make sure your portion size isn't excessive.

VEG VARIETY

Feel free to be as liberal with your veg as you like. Don't think that you need to restrict yourself to just one type of veg per meal, such as steamed broccoli with your chicken and rice. Instead, why not steam both green beans and broccoli, and grill some onion, pepper and courgette with your chicken? If you find vegetables boring, liven them up by adding herbs and spices. A bit of paprika with your mixed grilled vegetables, for example, will make them taste delicious.

DOUBLE DINNER

Making an extra protein portion with your evening meal is a great way of ensuring that you have a nutritious lunch for the next day. If you're having chicken or steak, for example, cook an extra portion and use it in a simple salad.

HEALTHY DINNER EXAMPLES

- Paprika grilled chicken and veg with new potato and steamed green beans
- Pan-fried steak with mashed potato, garlic mushrooms and tomato
- Soy-grilled salmon with vegetable rice and broccoli
- Home-made cheese burger with tomato and onion and a green side salad
- Home-made prawn and vegetable curry and rice

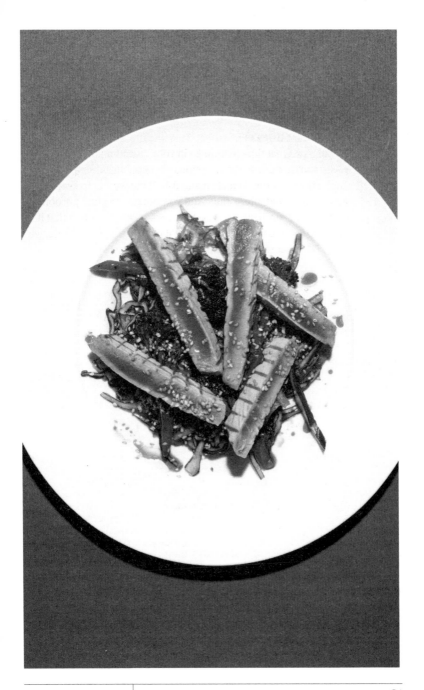

Healthy snacks

Here's what to eat between meals

Snacks often get overlooked when someone is thinking about creating a healthy diet. They usually focus their attention on the main meals and don't put much thought into what they'll eat between those meals. But eating conventional snacks, such as crisps and chocolate bars can quickly undermine your progress elsewhere. If you have a few healthy go-to options you won't resort to reaching for the biscuit tin.

There are a couple of other reasons why snacks can be helpful. They can fill in hunger gaps between meals, meaning that you don't ever get really hungry. That's good because its when you're starving that you tend to make poor food choices. They can also be portable, so you can carry them around with you. That kind of preparation means you won't get caught out when you're on the go. Here are a few simple and tasty options.

Protein shakes
You can buy these in ready-to-drink bottles or you can carry around some protein powder in a shaker and add water whenever you like. They're a really convenient way of getting a solid 30g protein hit, especially when your nutrition options are limited.

Beef jerky
This can be something of an acquired taste but the dried beef snacks are very useful because they can be left in your bag and used whenever required. Quality does tend to vary, and some have flavourings that contain added sugar, so our advice is to go for the best quality product available.

Natural yogurt
This is a protein-rich option that can also satisfy a craving for something desert-like, particularly if you eat it with some fruit. Just be aware that not all yogurts are created equally. Natural yogurt is great but fruit yogurts are usually packed with sugar.

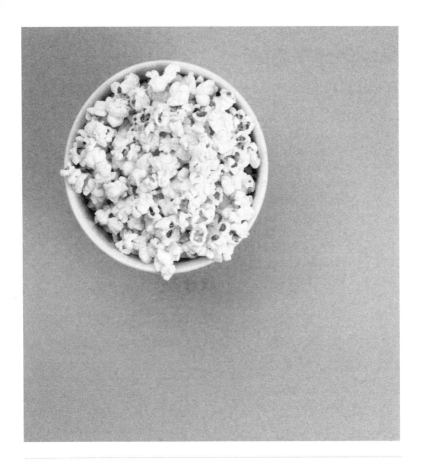

Nuts

Nuts such as brazils, walnuts and almonds contain healthy fats and a host of other useful nutrients. You do have to be aware that they are also quite calorific, so you want to make sure that your portion size is small. Rotating the nuts you eat, as opposed to always eating the same type, will help you to broaden your nutrient intake.

Popcorn

We've included this more as an alternative to crisps rather than because of its intrinsic nutritional merits. A serving of popcorn will have about half of the number of calories as a serving of crisps. So if you're struggling with your diet and you're craving foods you're trying to avoid, then it could be a tactical way to keep things on track.

Dark chocolate

Again, we're not saying that dark chocolate is amazing (although it does contain some health benefits). We're suggesting that you eat a couple of squares of dark chocolate rather than guzzling down a bar of milk chocolate. The dark variety contains much less sugar than other options.

Supplements

Your instant guide to the most popular supplements

WHEY PROTEIN POWDER
Whey protein is popular because it is rapidly digested and absorbed by your digestive system and so it gets into your muscles very quickly when consumed after training. This kick-starts the process known as muscle protein synthesis, where the amino acids in protein are used to rebuild and repair the muscular damage caused by weight training. It's not essential to consume whey protein powder because you should be able to get an adequate supply of protein from your diet, but it is a great convenient option if accessing good quality fresh food is difficult.

OMEGA-3
Omega-3 is an 'essential' fatty acid, which means we need to consume it directly from our diet. Good sources of Omega-3 include oily fish, nuts and seeds. Even though Omega-3 is a fatty acid, it has been shown to have a positive impact on fat loss as well as positively impacting brain function, inflammation levels and cardiovascular health. You can get your Omega-3 supply through your diet but because of the mercury levels found in some fish it may be safer to eat a couple of portions of fish a week and top yourself up with an Omega-3 supplement.

BCAAS
Branch-chain amino acids are a combined form of three of the nine essential amino acids: leucine, isoleucine and valine. They are called 'essential' amino acids because your body can't manufacture them itself from other compounds, so they must be taken in via the food you eat. Research has shown that BCAAs can improve muscular endurance, increase energy levels, and reduce recovery time. In short, they can help you train harder for longer. They can, however, deplete levels of other nutrients, such as vitamin B6, so if you're going to use BCAAs then you may want to consider a formulation that contains vitamin B6 or also taking a separate vitamin B6 supplement.

CREATINE

Creatine is useful for anyone who wants to increase their strength
and power. It can be synthesised by your body via your diet but
not in a significant quantity, which is why supplementation can be
useful. It is one of the best-researched supplements available and
has strong evidence to suggest that it is effective. Recent research
has shown that creatine can help your muscles work harder for
longer, so it's well worth considering if you're going to embark on
a period of intense strength training.

MULTIVITAMIN

Theoretically, if you're eating a wide variety of fresh, nutrient-
dense food then you won't need a multivitamin. It can, however,
be used as a bit of a safety net to ensure that if there are any gaps
in your nutrition intake then you have them covered. Of course,
some multi-vitamins contain relatively low levels of some key
nutrients, which reduces their effectiveness.

VITAMIN D

Vitamin D plays an essential role in a huge number of biological
and metabolic functions, as well as improving cognition, and
reducing the risk of certain cancers, cardiovascular disease and
dementia. It is produced by your body when your skin is exposed
to sunlight, but is also found in limited quantities in some foods,
such as fish and eggs. If you live in a country that doesn't get
much sun, such as the UK, then you should consider using a
supplement, particularly during the winter months. Be aware that
taking high doses can be toxic, because your body won't flush out
excess levels. It can also deplete levels of other essential nutrients,
such as vitamin K.

MAGNESIUM

In short, magnesium is essential in the process of energy
production and is found in nuts, green leafy vegetables and whole

grains. It is also integral to healthy nervous system function and has anecdotally been shown to improve sleep quality. It's probably worth experimenting with to see if you experience a benefit in that area, and also because intense exercise can leave your levels depleted.

ZINC

Zinc is involved in a huge number of biological roles, including DNA metabolism, gene expression, hormone production and function (including testosterone function), brain health, and central nervous system function. Shellfish and red meat, especially beef, lamb and liver, are the best dietary sources. It is possible to consume sufficient quantities of zinc through your diet but it can be lost in sweat, so if you're undertaking a high-intensity resistance training programme then it may be worth investing in supplementation. You can also get zinc combined with magnesium and vitamin B6 in a supplement called ZMA.

PRE-WORKOUT

Designed to be taken around 30 minutes before your training session, pre-workout supplements contain a combination of ingredients that claim to improve your gym performance. Because the ingredients vary from one product to another, it is hard to say categorically whether they are useful or not. Equally, some ingredients have better evidence to support them than others. For example, there is strong evidence to suggest that beta alanine can improve power endurance by buffering lactic acid. You should be aware that most products contain caffeine, so if you are sensitive to stimulants, or you exercise in the afternoon or the evening, then they may not be the best option.

CASEIN PROTEIN POWDER

This is a slow-digesting form of protein, which is why it is commonly used before bed. If you do consume it that way the amino acids are drip-fed to your muscles throughout the night. Like whey, it is found in dairy products, including cow's milk. It's probably not essential for beginners, or for those who are trying to lose fat. But if you're more advanced and you're trying to bulk up, it could be a useful weapon in your muscle building arsenal.

Quickfire supplement Q&A

We answer common supplement questions

Do I need supplements? Most supplements aren't essential, because you can obtain the relevant nutrients through your diet. But they can be convenient, such as drinking a post-workout protein shake. They can also, as in the case of a multivitamin, provide a nutritional safety net. Some nutrients, vitamins and minerals such as vitamin D3 and creatine are difficult to obtain in sufficient quantities through diet or lifestyle alone, which is why you might want to consider using a supplement.

Are supplements safe? The vast majority of supplements sold by reputable retailers are perfectly safe but if you want to get further reassurances that what's on the ingredient list is what's in the supplement then you should look for products with quality control assurances, such as an endorsement from Informed Sport, who test products for WADA-banned substances.

Are there any side effects? If you stick to the recommended dosage then it is unlikely that you will experience any side effects. However, some products, such as pre-workout formulas, contain substance such as caffeine, which you may be sensitive to. Other products, such as whey protein powder, may contain substances that you're intolerant of. For that reason, you should always carefully read the label before using any supplement.

Can I take supplements if I follow a special diet? Again, you'll need to read the label to make sure that a supplement satisfies your special diet. Some supplements where the active ingredient may not pose any issues are contained within casing that can be problematic. Not all supplements are vegetarian or vegan friendly, for example.

Can supplements replace meals? Generally, we'd advise against using supplements to replace meals. The clue is in the name. They should supplement a diet, rather than constitute its substance. The most common supplements that are presented as meal replacements are shakes and bars but they can be low in some key nutrients, such as fibre and dietary enzymes. The best diets are ones that contain a wide variety of fresh food and are topped up with smart and judicious supplement use.

Part 3
Key exercises

Master the hypertrophy moves that matter

When you step into the gym you have hundreds, if not thousands, of potential exercises to choose from. So how do you select the right ones for your goals? To take the pressure off, it's worth understanding that it isn't the case that certain exercises are perfect and others are useless. There are often instances where a number of different exercises would be valid selections. But what you should aim to do is use moves that give you a big bang for your training buck. This becomes even more relevant when you're a beginner, because you have so much potential to exploit. It's almost impossible to see a situation where a beginner would be better off doing a small isolation exercise such as a wrist curl rather than a big compound (multi-joint) exercise. As you progress you will need to expand your repertoire of exercises but the ones we've selected in this chapter will take you a long way. And when you've mastered them you can begin to add in new exercises.

GEAR GUIDE
You'll notice that the exercises in this section tend to focus on using your bodyweight or dumbbells and barbells. That's because those items of kit, if we class your body as a training tool, are so versatile and effective. We do also look at other useful items of kit later in the chapter, but when it comes to mastering the basics, the tried-and-tested kit is where we think you should start.

Compound moves Q&A

What are compound moves?

Compound moves are exercises that work multiple muscle groups simultaneously, such as the bench press, which will develop the chest, arms and shoulders. They are also exercises that involve multi-joint movements.

Why are they important?

They are important for a couple of reasons. They will let you lift heavy weights, which in turn will have a positive impact on your strength and your body composition. They also tend to be more 'functional' than isolation exercises that target just one muscle group, such as the biceps. This is because they translate to real-world movements.

Why have you selected these exercises?

The exercises in this chapter have been selected because they provide the biggest bang for your training buck. You don't need to perform an endless variety of exercises to make massive improvements to your strength and body composition. You need to perfect the most important exercises and then aim to increase the weight you can lift and manipulate the key training variables to keep making progress.

Are they the only moves that matter?

Absolutely not. But they are the moves that we'd recommend spending time on because they will give you considerable return. There are other moves that you can do that are useful but you have to weigh up the time it takes to learn these moves with the benefit that they'll provide. Our advice is to learn the exercises in this chapter and when you have built an appreciable ability in all of them then you can get more adventurous.

How do I know what weight to use?

This requires a bit of trial and error. But essentially whenever you're lifting a weight, you should aim to select one that allows you to only just complete all of the reps in all of the sets in your workout with perfect form. If you fail way before that, you've selected a weight that's too heavy. If you cruise through your reps, you've chosen a weight that's too light. One thing you'll see in a lot of gyms is guys trying to lift a weight that's too heavy and using shoddy form to help them complete the reps. Using a heavy weight may make them feel good but it won't make them look good.

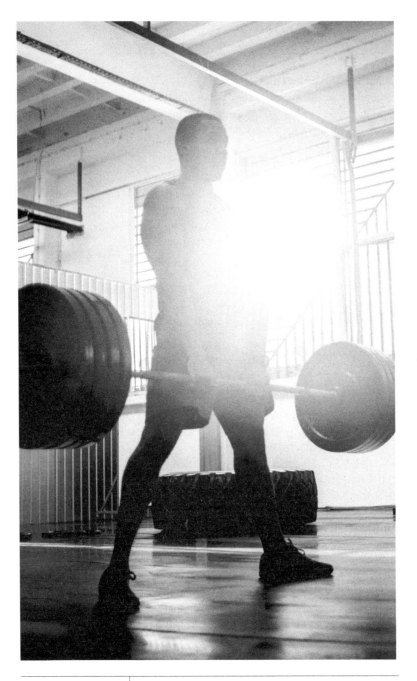

Key chest move: Bench press

Build a bigger chest with this classic barbell move

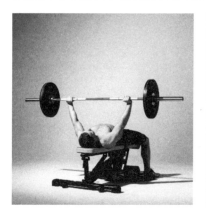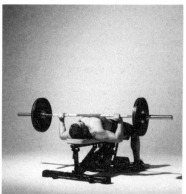

HOW TO DO IT

- Lie on a bench with your feet on the floor directly under or slightly behind your knees.
- Your head, upper back and glutes should be pressed hard against the bench.
- Hold the bar with an overhand grip, hands wider than shoulder-width apart.
- Before you initiate the movement, brace your core by contracting your abs and drawing your belly button in towards your spine.
- Slowly lower the bar under control until the bar is almost touching the middle of your chest.
- Make sure you use a full range of motion - avoid doing half reps.
- Pause at the bottom of the move to take the stretch reflex out of the lift and press back up hard to the start of the move, making sure you drive your feet into the floor.

WHY DO IT

This is one of the most popular barbell exercises and it is one that every guy wants to excel in. It's also excellent for developing upper-body muscular size, power and strength. It predominantly works the chest muscles but it also recruits the muscles at the front of the shoulders and the back of the arms (triceps), meaning that it will help you to build a bigger, more muscular upper body.

Best of the rest

CLOSE-GRIP BENCH PRESS

Why do it
Bringing your hands closer together moves the focus of the move away from the chest and to the triceps.

How to do it
- Lie flat on a bench holding a barbell with a close, overhand grip.
- Your grip should be either shoulder-width or just narrower than shoulder width apart.
- There should also be a small gap between your lower back and the bench.
- Before you initiate the movement, brace your core by contracting your abs and drawing your belly button in towards your spine.
- Lower the bar under control to your chest, keeping your elbows close in to your sides to keep the emphasis on your triceps.
- Push back up powerfully, making sure you drive your feet into the floor.

INCLINE BENCH PRESS

Why do it
Setting the bench to an incline will mean you need to reduce the weight, but it'll provide a new challenge and will also help to build your upper chest and the front of your shoulders. It's a useful variation to throw in once you've mastered the conventional iteration of the bench press.

How to do it
- Lie on a bench set at a 30-45° incline, holding a bar over your chest with your grip just wider than shoulder width apart.
- Your head, upper back and glutes should be pressed hard against the bench.
- Before you initiate the movement, brace your core by contracting your abs and drawing your belly button in towards your spine.
- Lower the bar until it's nearly touching your chest, then press it back up, making sure you drive your feet into the floor.

TRICEPS DIP

Why do it
The triceps dip is a fantastic bodyweight exercise for building an athletic upper body. It will develop your chest as well as your triceps and your front shoulders. It is, however, a very challenging exercise because you're moving the entire weight of your body, so you need to make sure that your shoulders are injury-free. It's also not one for beginners so it pays to build an appreciable level of strength in your chest and arms before you include it in your training regime.

How to do it
- Grip the bars, with your body upright.
- Before you initiate the movement, brace your core by contracting your abs and draw your belly button in to your spine.
- With your elbows pointing straight back, lower your body as far down as you can comfortably go without stressing your shoulders.
- Try to avoid swinging your legs for momentum.

Key legs move: Back squat

Add size and strength with the king of the legs moves

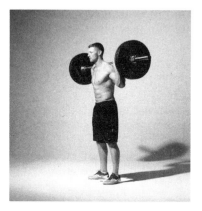 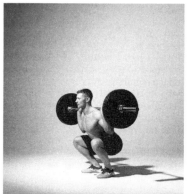

HOW TO DO IT

- Rest the bar on your upper back, rather than your neck, and hold it with an overhand grip slightly wider than shoulder-width apart.
- Your feet should be just wider than shoulder-width apart with your toes pointing outwards slightly.
- Before you initiate the movement, brace your core by contracting your abs and drawing your belly button in to your spine.
- Start the movement by simultaneously bending at the hips and the knees, keeping your chest and chin up throughout the rep.
- Keep the weight on your heels and your midfoot and don't let your knees fall inwards.
- Lower until your thighs are at least parallel to the floor.
- Drive back up through your heels, making sure you don't tip forwards or shift your weight onto your toes.

WHY DO IT

The barbell back squat is arguably the most important legs move that you can do. It not only works the quads but also the glutes, hamstrings, core and back. Because of the number of muscle groups involved in the exercise, you will be able to lift a substantial amount of weight once you perfect the technique.

Best of the rest

FRONT SQUAT

Why do it
Resting the bar on the front of your shoulders targets your quads while taking emphasis off your lower back. Even though we'd advise you to master the back squat first, the front squat is, in some respects, an easier exercise to master. On the other hand, some people struggle to get into position where the bar is resting on their upturned palms. If that's the case, you can use the cross-body technique described below.

How to do it
- Rest the bar on the front of your shoulders, with hands crossed in front of you.
- Brace your core by contracting your abs and drawing your belly button in to your spine.
- Lower until your thighs are at least parallel to the floor.
- Drive back up through your heels, making sure you don't tip forwards or shift your weight onto your toes - keeping your elbows up throughout the rep.

ROMANIAN DEADLIFT

Why do it
It is a version of the deadlift but it is much easier to learn. It's also much easier to do safely, if you stick to the form guide, and it will have the effect of generally helping to keep you injury-free because it will improve your posture.

How to do it
- Stand upright with your feet shoulder-width apart, holding a barbell with an overhand grip just outside your hips.
- Keep your shoulder blades retracted and your torso upright.
- Brace your core by contracting your abs and drawing your belly button in to your spine.
- Start the move by hinging at the hips, not the waist, and lower the bar slowly down the front of your legs until you feel a strong stretch in your hamstrings.
- Reverse the move and push your hips forward to return to the start.

BARBELL LUNGE

Why do it
The lunge is a single-leg exercise, so your body - and particularly your core - needs to work really hard to stay stable. This means that it is good for building strength, stability and athleticism. It does the latter because it develops something called proprioception - your body's ability to sense and respond to its own position.

How to do it
- Stand upright with a barbell resting on the back of your shoulders.
- Point your elbows down to retract your shoulder blades and keep your back upright throughout.
- Before you initiate the movement, brace your core by contracting your abs and drawing your belly button in to your spine.
- Take a big step forward, with your knee in line with your front foot.
- Lower until both knees are bent at 90°, then push back off your front foot to return to the start.

Key back move: Bent-over row

Develop a wider and thicker back with heavy rows

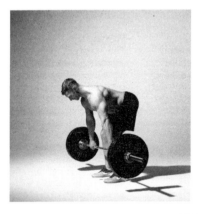 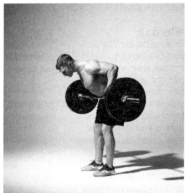

HOW TO DO IT

- Start with your back straight and your shoulder blades retracted.
- Bend your knees slightly and hinge at the hips.
- Grip the bar with your hands placed just wider than shoulder-width apart, letting the bar hang straight down.
- Before you initiate the movement, brace your core by contracting your abs and drawing your belly button in towards your spine.
- Pull the bar to your belly button, retracting your shoulder blades and almost trying to squeeze an imaginary orange between your shoulder blades to effectively contract the target back muscles.
- Lower the bar under control before starting the next rep.

WHY DO IT

If you want to build the perfect physique then you need to build a balanced physique. That means doing a roughly equal amount of chest (pressing) moves and back (pulling) moves. This exercise works the opposite muscle groups to the ones that you work during the bench press - the upper back (traps, lats, rhomboids and rear deltoids) - as well as your biceps and your abs, which will help to keep your torso stable.

Best of the rest

LAT PULLDOWN

Why do it
This works similar muscles to the pull-up but because you're performing the movement on a machine you can adjust the resistance easily. That means you can assess your progress but it also makes it an accessible exercise. Once you can perform multiple reps using your bodyweight you should be able to crank out a few pull-ups.

How to do it
- Sit on the seat and adjust the machine according to the instructions.
- Take an overhand, wide grip.
- Pull the bar down in front of you until it reaches your upper chest.
- Don't lean back to aid the movement because this will take tension off the target muscles.
- Aim to bring your elbows down to your sides to properly engage the back muscles.
- Squeeze your lats at the bottom of the move and return the bar slowly to the top.

PULL-UP

Why do it
The pull-up is a really challenging exercise because you have to lift up and control your entire bodyweight. If you're not able to do a single rep then you could try an eccentric rep, which just involves the lowering phase of the exercise. You jump up to top position then lower as slowly as you can. If you practise that for a while then you'll be able to transition to performing full reps.

How to do it
- Grip the bar with an overhand grip with your hands wider than shoulder-width apart.
- Start from a dead hang position with your arms straight.
- Before you initiate the movement, brace your core by contracting your abs and drawing your belly button in towards your spine.
- Pull yourself up then, once your chin is over the bar, pause briefly then slowly lower yourself back to the start.

CHIN-UP

Why do it
This exercise is very similar to the pull-up but it involves taking an underhand grip, with your palms facing towards you. That emphasises the role of the biceps so it's an essential tool in your arm-building arsenal. You'll also recruit the muscles of the back, helping you to build a strong upper body.

How to do it
- Grip the bar with an underhand grip with your hands shoulder-width apart.
- Start from a dead hang with your arms straight.
- Before you initiate the movement, brace your core by contracting your abs and drawing your belly button in towards your spine.
- Pull yourself up then, once your chin is over the bar, pause briefly then slowly lower yourself back to the start.

Key shoulder move: Shoulder press

Get broader shoulders with overhead presses

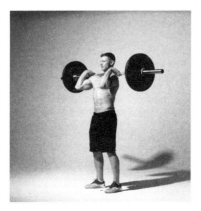 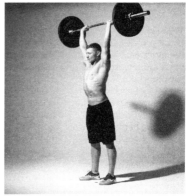

HOW TO DO IT

- With your feet shoulder-width apart, position a bar on your upper chest, gripping it with hands just wider than shoulder-width apart.
- Keep your chest upright and, before you initiate the movement, brace your core by contracting your abs and drawing your belly button in towards your spine.
- Press the bar directly overhead until your arms are straight.
- Lower the bar back to just below chin height - if you lower the bar further than that then you're likely to put an excessive amount of stress on your shoulder joint.

WHY DO IT

Pressing a heavy weight overhead will also build a rock-solid core because it takes huge effort to control the weight when it is overhead. The improved shoulder stability that it generates is also likely to give your bench press a boost too. It mainly targets the front and middle shoulders, so you'll need to also do some isolation work that targets your rear shoulders.

Best of the rest

PUSH PRESS

Why do it
Using your legs to initiate the move enables you to lift more weight and prevents poor form at the start of each rep (rounding your back, for example). Ensure you lower the bar back down to your shoulders slowly and under control to hit the muscles hard.

How to do it
- With your feet shoulder-width apart, position a bar on your upper chest.
- Before you initiate the movement, brace your core by contracting your abs and drawing your belly button in to your spine.
- Bend your knees slightly to lower into a quarter squat then stand back up explosively while pressing the bar overhead by straightening your arms.
- Lower the bar back to just below chin height - if you lower the bar further than that then you're likely to put an excessive amount of stress on your shoulders.

LANDMINE

Why do it
This is a great functional move because it requires control of the shoulder joint and it will help to build rotational strength, which is useful for sports movements. You also work one side at a time, which will help to build a balanced physique.

How to do it
- Wedge a barbell into a weight plate or the corner of the room so that it is fixed in position.
- Before you initiate the movement, brace your core by contracting your abs and drawing your belly button in towards your spine.
- Hold one end of the bar by your shoulder then press it up by straightening your arm.
- Lower the bar back to the start under control before repeating the exercise.

UPRIGHT ROW

Why do it
This exercise will help you to build wide shoulders, which will give you an impressive V-shaped torso appearance. It will also add size to your traps, the muscles of your upper back which give the impression of real strength.

How to do it
- Hold a bar on the front of your thighs with your hands just narrower than shoulder width apart.
- Before you initiate the movement, brace your core by contracting your abs and drawing your belly button in towards your spine.
- Pull the bar up to the top of your chest, leading with your elbows to focus the effort on your middle shoulders and traps.
- Lower the bar back to the start under control before repeating the exercise.

Key whole-body move: Deadlift

Get a whole-body workout with one move

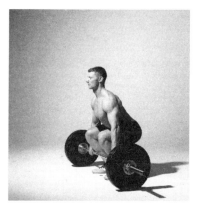 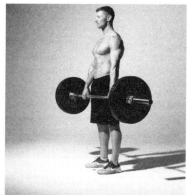

HOW TO DO IT

- Stand with your feet shoulder-width apart, grasping the bar with an overhand grip with your hands just outside your legs.
- Before you initiate the movement, brace your core by contracting your abs and drawing your belly button in towards your spine.
- Make sure there is tension in the hamstrings before you start the move then begin to straighten your legs without altering the angle of your torso.
- Once the bar is passed knee height you can begin to straighten your torso.
- Squeeze your glutes hard at the top but avoid pushing your hips too far forwards because that will stress your lower back.
- Lower the bar by reversing the movement - at no point should you ever round your lower back.

WHY DO IT

The deadlift is one of the most important exercises you can perform because of the sheer number of muscle groups that it uses. It is also excellent at working your entire posterior chain - the muscles on the back of your body. That's important because most guys tend to focus on the front of the body because those are the muscles that you can see in the mirror.

Best of the rest

POWER CLEAN

Why do it
This version of the full clean won't allow you to use as much weight, but it's much easier and safer to learn, so you can get on with your workout and use it to build serious explosive power, which is useful on the sports field and for targeting fast-twitch muscle fibres.

How to do it
- Stand with your feet shoulder-width apart, grasping the bar with an overhand grip with your hands just outside your legs.
- Start the move as if you were performing a deadlift but as the bar reaches mid-thigh height, push your hips through as explosively as possible to 'bang' the bar with your legs and drive it up.
- As the bar continues to rise, drop under it slightly to 'catch' it with upturned palms.
- Keep your elbows up to avoid dropping the bar.
- Stand up straight then drop the bar before re-setting.

FARMER'S WALK

Why do it
The farmer's walk is an excellent functional exercise, which will give you real-world benefits while building a strong grip and an iron core. You can perform farmer's walks with a variety of kit. Kettlebells are a great place to start because the relatively high handle makes it easy to pick the weights up off the floor.

How to do it
- Place a kettlebell just outside of both feet.
- Get into position as if you were going to deadlift the kettlebells.
- Pick the kettlebells up as if you were doing a deadlift.
- Once you have braced your core you can start to walk forwards.
- Aim to make your steps slow and con-trolled and avoid getting pulled out of position.
- If you're including a turn in your walk, make sure you do so under complete control.
- When you put the weights down, do so with control.

THRUSTER

Why do it
This exercise combines a front squat with an overhead press so it is seriously demanding. It therefore helps to build strength and also torch an enormous number of calories. You just need to make sure that as you get tired your form doesn't suffer. The main thing to watch out for is rounding your lower back as you squat down.

How to do it
- Holding a barbell with a shoulder-width grip. Squat down until your thighs are parallel to the floor.
- Before you initiate the movement, brace your core by contracting your abs and drawing your belly button in to your spine.
- Squat down and aim to lower until your thighs are parallel to the floor.
- Drive up explosively, using momentum to help press the bar overhead.
- Lower the bar to your chest and go straight into the next rep.

Isolation exercises

Use these exercises to build targetted muscle

Isolation exercises are ones that involve a single muscle group and a single joint, such as the triceps and the elbow joint in a triceps press-down. Now, there's sometimes a bit of snobbery about isolation exercises in some parts of the training world. They can be looked down on as 'vanity' exercises that are inferior to the tough, character-building compound lifts. Well, there's really only one sensible question to ask yourself: What's the best training tool for your goal? If the answer is a specific isolation move, then do that move. For instance, if you want bigger biceps and you've been doing heavy barbell bent-over-rows to grow your arms, that's great. But what happens when your big back muscles fatigue and you can't do any more reps? Your biceps aren't strong enough to move the bar on their own so the set ends before your biceps have been fatigued. In this instance, it may be wise to throw in some direct biceps exercises to properly fatigue the muscles.

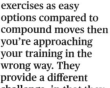

DON'T GO EASY
If you think of isolation exercises as easy options compared to compound moves then you're approaching your training in the wrong way. They provide a different challenge, in that they don't generally excite your central nervous system in the same way that compound moves do. But you should still focus on giving absolutely everything you've got when you do an isolation move and if you think they're easy you're not working hard enough.

Chest exercises

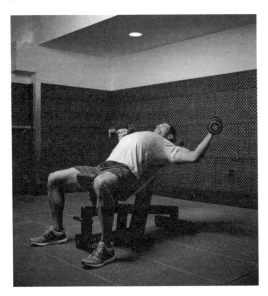

CABLE CROSSOVER

Why do it

It's hard to truly isolate your powerful chest muscles - the arms and shoulders nearly always get in on the act because of the way your upper body muscles move together. But this move is a great way to work the chest because using cables, rather than dumbbells, for resistance ensures that there is constant tension throughout the move, which forces your chest to work hard to control the weight.

How to do it

- Stand in the middle of a cable machine with a split stance, holding a D-handle attachment in each hand and with the cable set above shoulder height.
- Keeping a natural arch in your back, your core braced and your upper body still, bring your hands down in an arc to meet in front of your torso.
- Pause briefly and squeeze your chest muscles, then return to the start slowly and with the weight under full control.

DUMBBELL FLYE

Why do it

This move isolates your chest muscles, taking your arms out of the equation so all the work has to be done by your chest. It's a great move to use as a second exercise in a superset with a bench press variation. It can also be paired with a reverse flye in an antagonistic superset.

How to do it

- Lie on an incline bench holding a dumbbell in each hand directly above your chest, with arms straight and palms facing each other.
- Make sure your head and shoulders are supported on the bench and your feet are flat on the floor.
- With a slight bend in your elbows, slowly lower the weights out to the side as far as is comfortable.
- Don't arch your back.
- Use your pecs to reverse the movement and raise the weights back to the top.

Biceps exercises

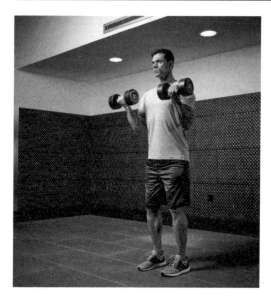

DUMBBELL BICEPS CURL

Why do it
The classic biceps exercise can be incredibly effective if done well. The key to executing it successfully is making sure that it's the target muscle, rather than the front shoulders or momentum, that does the work.

How to do it
- Stand upright with a dumbbell in each hand by your sides.
- Brace your core then initiate the movement by ever so slightly drawing your elbow back as you begin to bend your elbow. This will help to ensure that it is your biceps that do the bulk of the work.
- Raise the weights with your palms facing up until your forearms are vertical then squeeze the biceps muscle hard at the top of the rep.
- Lower slowly under control and squeeze your triceps before starting the next rep.

INCLINE BICEPS CURL

Why do it
By doing biceps curls on an incline bench, you move through a greater range of motion than when standing up, so it provides a different stimulus to your biceps.

How to do it
- Sit on a bench set on an incline between 30° and 45° holding a dumbbell in each hand.
- Keeping your back flat against the bench and your elbows close to your sides, slowly curl the dumbbells up to shoulder height.
- Squeeze your biceps at the top of the rep then slowly return to the start.

Triceps exercises

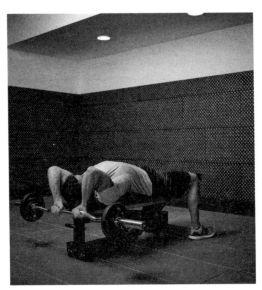

LYING EZ-BAR TRICEPS EXTENSION

Why do it
This move works to isolate your triceps, forcing the muscle to work hard throughout as you control the weight on the way down before raising it again. Start by using a light weight because you need to manage the weight safely as you lower it towards your head.

How to do it
- Lie flat on a bench, holding an EZ-bar above you with straight arms.
- Slowly lower the bar towards the top of your head by bending your elbows, which should point upwards throughout the move.
- Try to avoid your elbows flaring out to the side because that will take tension off the target muscle.
- Without arching your back, return the bar to the start position.

CABLE TRICEPS PRESS DOWN

Why do it
The advantage of using a cable machine is that it provides resistance throughout the whole move, forcing your triceps to work hard to manage the weight on the way up as well as on the way down. Keep your elbows close to your sides so that the emphasis stays on your triceps.

How to do it
- Stand tall at a cable machine with a double rope handle or straight bar handle attached at head height.
- Keeping your elbows tucked in, press the handle down without rocking forwards.
- Squeeze your triceps at the bottom of the move, then slowly return to the start.

Back exercises

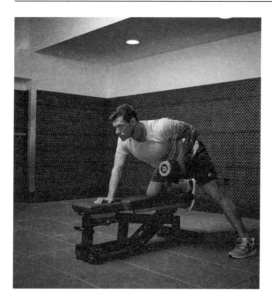

SINGLE-ARM ROW

Why do it
A lot of people struggle to properly contract their big back muscles because they struggle to 'feel' them working. That can particularly be the case with bent-over rows. You also often see that exercise done badly, with a lot of torso movement and a poor range of motion. With single arms rows, you can really focus on pulling your elbow back and feeling the target lat muscles contracting.

How to do it
- Rest your left knee and left hand on a bench, holding a dumbbell in your right hand close to the floor.
- Keeping your back straight, use your back muscles and biceps to row the weight up to your side, leading with your elbow.
- Rather than thinking of the movement path as a straight line, you may find it more effective to think of it as an arc. That will help you to really contract the target muscle.
- Repeat the move on the other side.

STRAIGHT-ARM CABLE PULLDOWN

Why do it
Standing up and keeping your arms straight fully engages the lats and prevents your biceps - or any other back muscles - and momentum getting in on the act. Just make sure that you start with your shoulders down, to prevent your traps aiding the movement. Also make sure that your arms are straight. It's really easy to keep a slight bend in the arms and let your triceps take over at the end of the rep. This isn't a move where you'll shift heavy weights so don't worry if you need to go light.

How to do it
- Stand tall in front of a cable machine with a straight bar attached to the top pulley.
- Holding the bar with an overhand grip, pull it down until it reaches the top of your thighs, keeping your arms straight throughout.
- Slowly return to the start.

Shoulder exercises

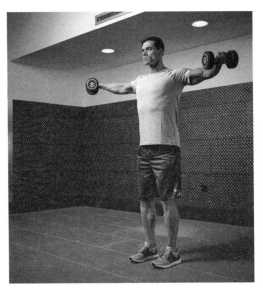

REVERSE FLYE

Why do it
This is a great move for targeting the muscles that make up the rear part of your shoulders. It's often neglected in favour of working the other shoulder muscles, but you need balanced growth to ensure that you get wide shoulders. You can either do it while bent over at the hips or you can do it prone on a bench. Both are good options. Just make sure you don't go too heavy because lifting a load that's too heavy is a sure-fire way of involving other muscles that you didn't intend to use.

How to do it
- Lie flat on a bench, holding a dumbbell in each hand.
- Keeping a slight bend in your elbows, raise the weights out to the sides until they're at shoulder height, then return to the start.

LAT RAISE

Why do it
This is a brilliant isolation exercise but you often see people doing it incorrectly. When you start the move, you want to initiate the movement using your side delts, not your traps, so keep your shoulders down throughout the exercise to make sure you use good technique. Avoid raising the weights above shoulder height because this may stress the shoulder joint, which can be a very delicate joint, and will provide minimal muscle-gain benefit. Finally, imagine you're pouring a glass of water as you lift - that will ensure that you lead with your little finger.

How to do it
- Stand holding a dumbbell in each hand on the outside of your thighs.
- Initiating the movement using your middle delts, raise both arms up to your sides, leading with the little finger on each hand.
- Raise the dumbbells to shoulder height then lower them under control, rather than letting gravity take over.

Quads exercises

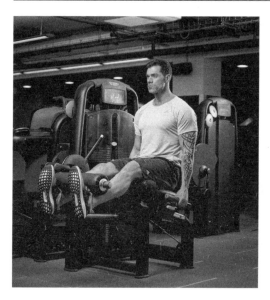

LEG EXTENSION

Why do it
This is a classic quad-builder and it is very popular with bodybuilders because it is so effective at adding size. The benefit of machines is that you can go to failure comparatively safely because your movement path is fixed. If you collapse under a heavy barbell back squat, you could be in trouble but machine exercises are a good way of pushing the target muscle. That's not an excuse to get sloppy and use poor form, however - you still need to use good technique.

How to do it
- Sit in the leg extension machine, making sure your back is resting against the back rest.
- Adjust the pad so it sits on top of your shins just above your feet.
- Hold the handles for stability and contract your quads to move the weight stack.
- Fully contract your quads, squeezing the muscles at the top of the rep then lower slowly under control.

BULGARIAN SPLIT SQUAT

Why do it
This is a really underused exercise. It's excellent at isolating the quads while providing a real test of balance and stability. You don't need to go heavy to make this move challenging and because it is unilateral (one-sided) it will help you to balance out your strength.

How to do it
- Place one foot on a bench behind you with your other foot slightly in front of you. Load via dumbbell or kettlebell in each hand if required.
- Squat down through the front leg, keeping the foot flat on the ground and rear leg bent. Ensure that the knee does not crash into the floor.
- Drive up evenly through the front foot, ensuring it remains flat on the floor at all times. Do not tip forwards onto the toes.

Hamstring exercises

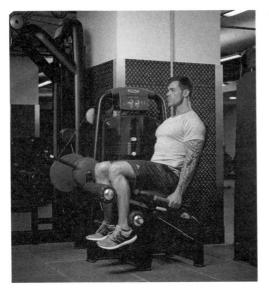

GLUTE/HAM RAISE

Why do it
In truth, this isn't really an isolation move because it will work your glutes as well as your hamstrings, but it's so effective that we had to include it. It's great because it develops key muscles in your posterior chain - the ones on the back of your body that most guys could do with spending more time on.

How to do it
- Position yourself in a glute/ham raise machine with your knees behind the pad and toes driven into the foot plate.
- Brace your core, contract your glutes and lower slowly under control.
- Whilst staying in complete control of your movement, lower until your legs are straight, keeping the torso rigid. Return to upright by driving the toes into the foot plate and contracting your hamstrings, glutes and even your calves.

HAMSTRING CURL

Why do it
Like the leg extension for your quads, this is the classic machine exercise for your hamstrings. Some machines involve lying face down and curling the weight up. Others will have you sitting down to perform the move. Whatever way they are set up, they will effectively isolate the hamstrings and let you really hone in on that muscle. Machines like this are also useful for doing drop sets because you can adjust the resistance quickly without needing a training partner.

How to do it
- Set up the machine so that the pads sit comfortably against your lower back when you sit on it.
- Put your legs on the padded lever so it sits just below your calf muscles, and set up the lap pad so it sits on your thigh just above the knee.
- Grip the handles for stability then use your hamstrings to curl the bar down.
- Squeeze your hamstrings at the base of the move then return to the start under control.

Abdominal training

Why there's more to abs than hundreds of crunches

If you ask any guy what body part he'd most like to develop, there's a good chance that he'd go for a rock-solid six pack. A defined midsection is seen as the physique holy grail. Although the rectus abdominis - the sheet of muscle that makes up the six-pack - will be visible at different body fat percentages on different people, you can't have a visible six pack without having low levels of body fat.

Of course, it's not just the exercises you do that will determine how defined your abs are. You'll need to follow the advice in the nutrition chapter of this book if you want to reduce your belly fat so that your six-pack is visible.

It's also worth pointing out that a visible six-pack isn't the definitive signal that someone is in good shape. Those who prioritise strength may not feel that they need to reduce their body fat to a level where their abs are visible. They may even feel getting that lean will be detrimental to their strength goals. If you look at the typical World's Strongest Man competitor or an elite heavyweight powerlifter, you'll see phenomenal amounts of muscle but you may not see too many six packs.

If you are going to train your abs directly - and we recommend that you do if you want defined abs - then you have a huge amount of exercises to choose from. The list we've outlined over the following pages require varying levels of skill but they will target the different portions of the abs and will give you the training stimulus you're looking for. You need to do a variety of exercises to ensure that you hit these different areas. If, for example, you only ever did crunches, that would predominantly target the upper abs, which would mean you'd have underdeveloped lower abs and side abs. You also want to do exercises, such as the plank, that challenge the deep-lying muscles of the core that you can't see.

You can do a dedicated abs session but we suggest that a more efficient way to train is to add two or three exercises on to the end of your session. You don't want to do them at the start of a session because that's when you need your abs to be fresh so that they can stabilise your torso and maintain good posture during heavy compound moves, such as squats and deadlifts. If you lose abdominal control during a heavy squat you may crumple forwards and risk a disc injury. So leave them to the end for best results.

CRUNCH

How to do it: Lie on your back with your fingers by your temples and your knees bent with your feet flat on the floor. Exhale to contract your abs then, using your abdominal muscles, slowly curl your torso off the floor. It's more important to get a good contraction in your abs than it is to raise your torso really high off the floor. You also need to make sure that you don't pull your neck. Having your fingers by your temples, as opposed to having your hands clasped behind your head, will help you to do that. Pause briefly at the top then lower slowly under control rather than just dropping to the floor.

Why do it: This is a great exercise for developing your upper abs but so many people do it ineffectively. Our advice is to concentrate on quality of contraction and to keep your reps slow and controlled rather than banging out junk reps.

REVERSE CRUNCH

How to do it: Lie flat on your back with knees bent and arms flat against the floor.

Contract your lower abs to draw your knees in towards your chest. Pause at the top of the move and squeeze your abs, then return to the start.

Why do it: The standard crunch will develop your upper abs but this one will target your often-neglected lower abs, which you need to develop if you want a true six-pack.

CRUNCH REACH

How to do it: This is similar to a standard crunch but the difference is that you start with your arms straight and pointing up to the ceiling. As you crunch up, your arms should continue to reach up to the ceiling, as opposed to coming forwards. Lower under control and repeat the exercise.

Why do it: Keeping your hands in the air will ensure that the work needs to be done by your abs, rather than your hands forcing your head forwards and staining the neck. It's arguably easier to get and feel a good contraction in your abs doing this version of the crunch.

HANGING KNEE RAISE

How to do it: Hang from a pull-up bar with straight arms. Contract your abs then bend your knees and raise them up to hip height. Pause then lower them slowly under control before starting the next rep.

Make sure that you use your abs to power the move. It's really easy to let momentum take over and swing into and out of each rep but that won't do much to build your six-pack.

Why do it: This exercise will help to develop your lower abs, which can be quite hard to target when you're on the floor. Hanging from the bar will also provide a grip strength challenge, which will benefit other areas of your training.

HANGING LEG RAISE

How to do it: This is a progression from the hanging knee raise. In this move, you start in the same position as the hanging knee raise but instead of bending your knees, you raise your feet to hip height while keeping your legs straight. It's a tough exercise so it is worth perfecting the knee raise first before you progress to the leg raise.

Why do it: It's a tough move but it's an effective one because it places such a substantial demand on your abdominal muscles. But you can't cheat it. If you use momentum to assist your reps that may satisfy your ego but it won't do much to build your muscles.

PLANK

How to do it: This is one of the iconic abs exercises but, again, it's one that's often done poorly. To get into the correct start position, make sure that your body is in a straight line from head to heels and that your neck is in a neutral position, rather than looking forwards. Your elbows should be directly below your shoulders and your forearms should be flat on the floor. Draw your belly button in towards your spine to properly contract the abs and try to breathe as normally as possible without taking tension off your midsection. If your hips rise excessively, that will take tension off the abs and if they sag you'll stress your lower back. If you feel like your form is being compromised, bring the set to an end.

Why do it: This will not only target the outer abs but also the deep lying stabilising muscles that are so crucial for other big compound lifts such as squats and deadlifts.

BARBELL ROLLOUT

How to do it: Get an Olympic barbell ready by putting a large weight plate on either end. Kneel on the floor with your arms straight and your shoulders over the bar. Contract your abs and gradually roll the bar forwards. Go as far as you can while maintaining control of your midsection. If you can go all the way so that your nose is almost touching the floor, great. But if you can only go half that distance, it's more important that you maintain good

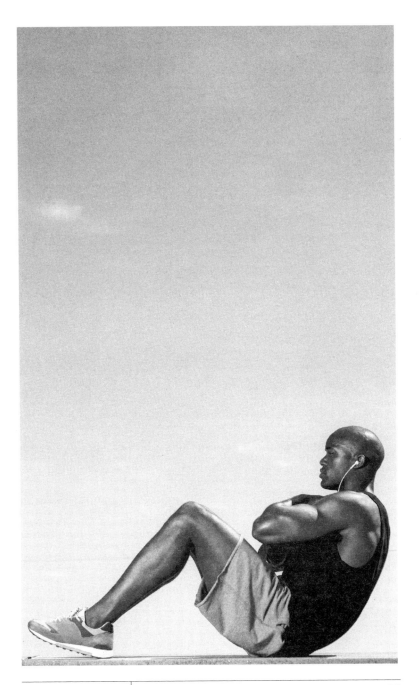

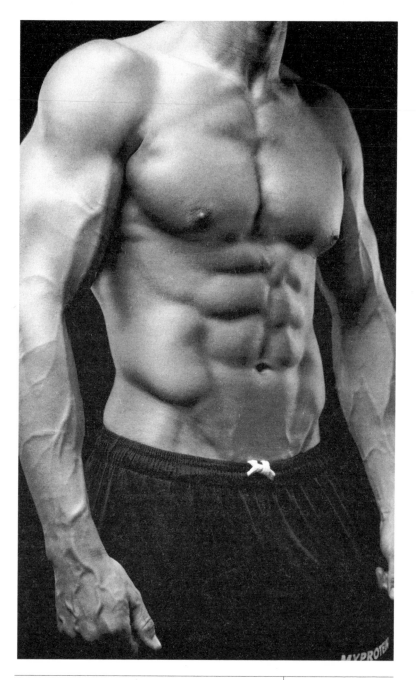

GET LEAN AND STRONG

technique than it is to compromise form while chasing range of motion. Once you've gone as far as you can go, return under control to the start. It may be harder to do the initial bit of the return portion of the exercise than it is to roll the bar out in the first place so bear that in mind while you're performing each rep.

Why do it: Some people consider this to be one of the most effective abs exercises you can do because it creates tension over such a large range of motion. But it's not easy, so we advise you to build a bit of abs strength first before you attempt it.

TURKISH GET-UP

How to do it: This exercise involves moving from lying to standing while holding a weight. A kettlebell is a convenient option because the handle is easy to hold but you could also use a dumbbell. Start by lying on the floor with your legs together and the weight in one hand above your shoulder. Bend your knee on the side that's holding the weight, keeping your foot flat on the floor. Place your free hand out to the side then contract your abs to raise your torso slightly off the ground and come up onto the elbow of your free hand. From there, push through your free hand to straighten your arm before bringing your straight leg back so you rest on your knee. Next, take your free hand off the floor to straighten your torso before standing up. Make sure that you keep the movement controlled and look at the load you're carrying throughout the move. Reverse the movement back to the start and repeat the exercise.

Why do it: This provides a huge test of core strength, co-ordination and stability. It also forces you to go from lying to standing, which is an almost unparalleled range of movement for an exercise.

INCREASING THE RESISTANCE

After you've been doing some of these bodyweight abs moves for a while you'll be able to do a number of reps that mean you're just training endurance rather than increasing muscle strength and size. There's little point in banging out 50 crunches, for example. So once you can do sets of 20, think about making the exercise harder by adding external resistance. For crunches, you can hold a weight plate or a dumbbell to your chest, for example. For exercises where it isn't easy to add load, such as the plank, you can do progressions of the exercise that make it harder. A decline plank, for example, where your feet are raised on a step, will increase the abdominal challenge. So too will a gym ball plank, where your forearms rest on a gym ball and you have to control the instability.

Bodyweight exercises

Burn fat and build muscle without any kit

Your body is arguably one of the most effective bits of exercise equipment available to you. We've already identified that pull-ups and chin-ups are excellent exercises for developing back and biceps size and strength and that the triceps dip is great for building chest and triceps strength. There are some in the training world who believe that you shouldn't attempt to use workout kit before you have mastered your own bodyweight. It's an interesting idea but there are flaws in the argument. An obese beginner may struggle to do a single press-up because they lack the strength and it may also put undue stress on their wrists. They may be better off doing some dumbbell bench presses first then progressing to press-ups. So you need to use bodyweight moves just as thoughtfully as you would any other type of exercise. Here are some others we recommend you try.

Key bodyweight moves

PRESS-UP VARIATIONS

The press-up is such an effective and versatile exercise but it is also one that's done really poorly. You need to make sure that you start the move in the right position, and that means your body is in a straight line from head to heels. If your hips rise that will take tension off the abs and if they sag that will place stress on the lower back. So get straight and get tight by pulling your belly button in towards your spine. Make sure your hands are level with your chest, not your face, and don't let your elbows flare out to the side. Use a proper range of motion and control the lowering phase before pressing back up powerfully. There are so many versions that you can do. If you want to target your triceps, do diamond press-ups. If you want to emphasise your chest, do wide press-ups. For increased shoulder strength and stability, try dive-bomber press-ups, and to build explosive power, do ballistic press-ups.

BODYWEIGHT VERSIONS

There's value to be gained by doing bodyweight versions of the exercises from earlier in this chapter. Bodyweight squats and lunges, for example, are great for developing leg strength, particularly if you're a beginner. You can also do them as the second move in a superset, for example, which will help you to fully and safely fatigue the target muscle. You can also use them as a primer ahead of a big move. Doing sets of fast bodyweight squats can fire up your central nervous system ahead of a heavy barbell squat set.

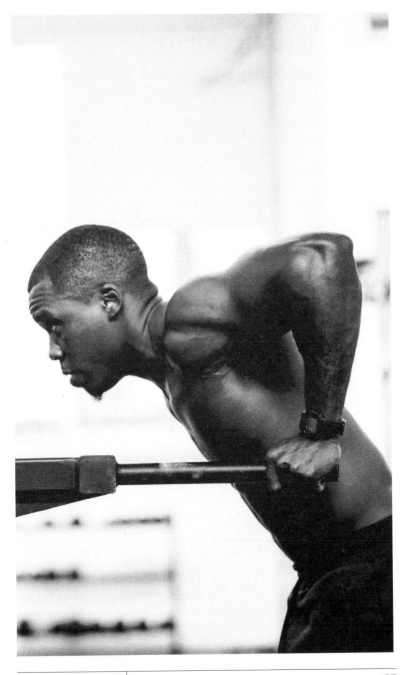

Other training kit

Expand your training horizons with this useful gear

MEDICINE BALLS

Medicine balls are really satisfying to use and they have two distinct benefits. You can use them to create instability, which will improve the strength of your stabilising muscles. You could do a press-up with one hand on the ball, for example. Their real value, however, comes in explosive moves, which you can use to either develop power or as an active warm-up to excite your central nervous system. Key explosive exercises include slams and throws, which are useful because you can go all-out. That's probably more appropriate for a beginner or an intermediate lifter than the Olympic lifts, which are much more technical and require you to master the deceleration phase. But with a slam, for example, you will instinctively know what to do. The other key bit of advice is to not worry too much about weight and instead concentrate on using maximum effort.

Key medicine ball moves

Overhead throw
You'll probably need to do this outside. Hold the ball in both hands, swing it between your legs, then explode upwards and throw it backwards over your head. Either retrieve the ball, get a friend to pass it back, or reset for the next rep.

Slam
Hold the ball in both hands, bring it behind your head and slam it to the floor as hard as possible. If you're focusing on cardio, retrieve the ball as fast as possible. If you're working on explosive-ness, reset between reps for maximum power.

Passing press-up
With one hand on the medicine ball, do a press-up. Keep your body in a straight line from neck to feet, and go as low as possible. At the top of the move, roll the ball across your body and put the other hand on it. Do another press-up. That's one rep.

BATTLE ROPES

Like medicine balls, battle ropes are really fun to use. They also give you a kind of cardiovascular challenge that it is difficult to get from traditional cardio kit such as treadmills, rowers and bikes because they pose a huge challenge to your upper body. Doing slams and waves will get your shoulders and biceps on fire in no time. And that's another huge benefit - they are so time efficient because they are so demanding. Doing just a few 20-second bursts of activity followed by a short rest will see you working at or near your maximum capacity.

Key battle rope moves

Slam
Hold a rope in each hand, raise both arms and then slam them down together, aiming to create a wave that travels all the way to the anchor point. For added cardio benefits, throw in a slight jump with each slam. You can also do this by alternating arms.

Biceps wave
Keeping the rest of your body still, wave the ropes as fast as possible, focusing on high reps and high amplitude. This move will see your biceps and grip affected by fatigue before your legs and lungs.

Lateral lunge
As you create ripples in the rope, perform a lateral lunge to one side, then the other. You'll bring your whole body into play, but also get some core work from keeping the ropes under control as you move.

Cardiovascular training

How to make the most of your cardio sessions

We've already established that steady-state jogging may not be the most efficient way to exercise if improving your body composition is your primary objective. That said, steady-state jogging isn't the only option available to you and there are a lot of health and fitness benefits to be derived from cardiovascular training, including mental as well as physical ones. These are the main types of cardio training that you can do, with the benefits and drawbacks of each one explained.

Running

Steady state jogging: It's not the most effective way to run but it's probably the easiest. And since running can be a mental battle (anyone who has laced up a pair of running shoes will be familiar with the voice in your head telling you to stop when you get tired) there's something to be said for making life easy. If you really love running and you find that it boosts your mood and clears your head, the odd steady state session (particularly if it is in the outdoors) can be a worthy addition to your programme.

Interval sessions: Interval running sessions are those where you combine periods of fast running with periods of slower recovery running. How you structure the sessions is entirely up to you and should be defined by your fitness levels and your overall goals. But in essence intervals are a good way of getting a lot of challenging work into a short session.

Tempo training: This is when you try to sustain a fast pace for an extended period of time. It should be around the pace that you can only just sustain and is likely to be a session that lasts about 20-30 minutes. It's designed to push your top cruising speed forwards and is another way of getting a good workout in a short period of time.

Sprinting: This is the most technically, physically and mentally challenging way to run, but it is also the method that will help you to build muscle as well as burn fat. You've only got to look at elite sprinters to see how good flat-out running can be for your physique. You should, however, be aware that sprinting will expose any weak strength links, particularly in your hamstrings. So we only advise you to do sprint sessions once you have an appreciable level of posterior chain strength and you make sure that you warm up thoroughly.

Hill running: Hill running is very tough but very effective. Obviously, the steeper the hill, the harder it is. One of the reasons we like it is because it provides a really big challenge but doesn't carry a high injury risk. You may want to run up and then walk or jog back down to recover. You can go fast down the hills too but that may stress your knee joints.

Trail running: This is off-road running and the uneven surface produces a unique challenge that will help to strengthen your connective tissue. A lot of people like trail running because of the wild environment and the unpredictable nature of the runs, with the benefit being both mental and physical.

Other cardio options

Cycling
One of the benefits of cycling is that is very low impact, so it's comparatively kind to your joints. The gear can be expensive but it also gives you the opportunity to cover ground and set off on adventures. Indoor cycling classes can be great for burning calories and torching fat.

Swimming
Swimming gives you a great full-body, low-impact workout. It does take you a while to develop an efficient technique but while your beginner-style thrashing around may not win any races, you can comfort yourself with the fact that your inefficiency is quite good for fat loss.

Indoor rowing
Indoor rowing will give you a great full-body workout and can be added to the end of a session to give you a fat loss 'finisher'. Just make sure that you pull with good technique. Excessively rounding your back when you start the stroke can put pressure on your back and cause injury.

Part 4
Training theory

The information you need to take charge of your workouts

Training theory is something that you could study for the rest of your life and still not fully exhaust all of the nuances and variations. There are, however, certain key concepts that will give you a solid foundation so that you can be the master of your own training destiny. And that's what your training efforts should be focused on: mastering the variables and protocols that give you the biggest bang for your buck. So, if we're to give you one overarching piece of advice it would this: concentrate on the big stuff. Get that right and you're ahead of most gym-goers. Once you've dealt with the basics, that's when you can get fancy. But if you dive in with the intricate and fussy stuff, you're missing the point. This chapter is devoted to giving you a guide to the most important training theory ideas for burning fat, building muscle and getting stronger. It is by no means an exhaustive treatment of the subject but it will stand you in good stead for the rest of your training career.

FOUNDATIONS FIRST
The reason we advise you to take on board the training theory basics before you start getting fancy is because they're the foundations of your progress. If you try to move on before you've built the foundations then you're going to be on shaky ground. The other thing that you should always keep in mind is that no fancy plan can replace effort and hard. If you want to make a difference to how you look and feel, you're going to have to roll your sleeves up and get to work.

Sample fat loss session

Here's what a fast, effective fat loss workout looks like

One of the simplest, most effective and most versatile approaches you can take to constructing a fat loss session is to do a simple barbell circuit. Using just one item of kit makes life easy because you can focus on executing the exercises rather than messing around getting your equipment ready. Circuits are essentially groups of exercises performed in a sequence with minimal rest. That's good for fat loss because the lack of rest will keep your heart rate up and it will maximise calorie burn, both during and after the session. Resistance-based circuits, like the one below, are also superior to pure cardio sessions because you will get a muscle-building effect, which you don't get from steady state running, for example. That means you'll not only lose fat but you'll also add some muscle, which will give you an athletic, cover-model physique, rather than just making you skinny.

Barbell super-circuit

How to do it:
Do 10 reps of each exercise in order, taking minimal rest between exercises, to complete one circuit. Rest for 90 seconds between circuits and complete 3-6 circuits. Start with an empty Olympic bar (20kg) and gradually add weight as your strength and fitness improves.

1. Romanian deadlift
Stand tall with a barbell resting on the front of your thighs. With a slight bend in your knees, push your backside back and hinge at the hips to send the bar down the front of your legs until you feel a strong stretch in your hamstrings. Return to the start and repeat.

2. Bent-over row
Start in the stretched position of the Romanian deadlift then contract your abs and pull the bar up to your belly button, leading with your elbows and keeping your torso angle stable. Lower the weight back down to the start and repeat.

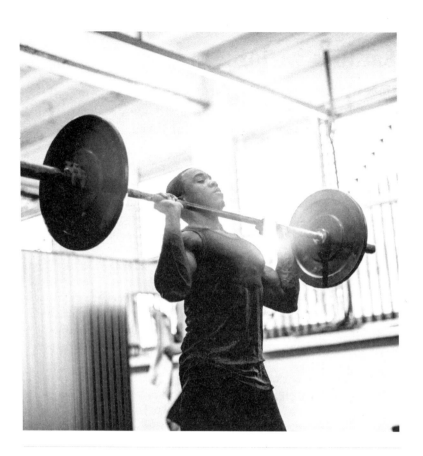

3. Hang clean
Perform the first half of a Romanian deadlift then powerfully stand up straight by bringing your hips through so that your thighs hit the bar and raise it to chest height. While it is still rising, drop into a half front squat to catch the bar on your shoulders with your palms facing up. Re-set and repeat.

4. Front squat
With the bar resting on the front of your shoulders, your palms facing up, simultaneously bend at the hips and knees to lower towards the floor until your thighs are parallel to the floor. Keep your weight on your heels and mid-foot and keep your torso upright. Return to the start and repeat.

5. Overhead press
After your final squat, drop your elbows so that they are below the bar then press the bar directly overhead until your arms are straight. Lower back down to the start and repeat. Make sure you don't lower the bar past your chin because that will stress your shoulder joint.

Fat loss variables

How to adjust your fat loss sessions

Length of session
First, the good news: fat loss sessions are typically shorter than muscle-building sessions. And here's the bad news: that's because they're supposed to be intense. That intensity will ensure you get a good calorie burn and you also get a solid cardio challenge. When it comes to adding size, it takes time to properly fatigue a muscle group, particularly if you're an advanced lifter. But with fat loss, you can get a really good workout in as little as four minutes. The Tabata method, for example, involves doing eight 20-second periods of work with 10-second rests in-between. Sounds easy, right? Well, it's probably the hardest workout you can do, because you're supposed to go at 100% for the entire thing. The majority of fat loss sessions probably take 20-40 minutes. If you're doing over an hour, it's unlikely you're working at the right intensity.

Number of exercises
There's probably more flexibility in this area for fat loss than there is for muscle-building. When it comes to building muscle if you do too few exercises you won't fatigue the target muscle group but if you do too many you'll end up doing lots of 'junk' reps with light weights. For fat loss, it's more about the effort and intensity level than it is about the number of exercises.

Fat loss session formats

Circuits: This is probably the simplest fat loss session that you can do. It's essentially a sequence of exercises performed back to back with no or minimal rest. Once you've completed one set of each move you then rest before going again.

Ladders: This involves a rep sequence that either increases or decreases. So, you may do 1 rep, rest for a short period and then do 2 and so on until you get to 10 reps. You can follow any number sequence you like. You could start at 5 and go up in 5. You can also pick two exercises, starst with 1 rep of the first move and 10 reps of the second. You then do 2 and 9 reps until you get to 10 and 1 reps.

Type of exercises

The thing that's more important than the number of exercises
is the type of exercise that you select. Generally you want to do
compound rather than isolation exercises because they will have
greater calorie-burn effect. It's tricky (but not impossible) to get
a real sweat on when you're doing biceps curls. It's certainly a lot
easier to give yourself a cardiovascular challenge while doing a
squat or lunge variation than it is by doing an isolation move that
targets the arms. One common way of including lots of compound
moves without completely battering yourself into the ground it to
alternate upper and lower body moves. That way half your body
gets to recover while the other half rests. If you just did moves
that focused on a couple of muscle groups, you'd fatigue too
quickly.

Work/rest ratio

Again, this is pretty fluid. But it is likely in a fat loss session that
your work periods will be greater than your rest periods. This
means you'll have to lift lighter weights than if you were doing
a hypertrophy or a strength session. The point is really finding
the right balance that allows you to complete as much work as
possible and as high an intensity as you can manage.

AMRAP: For fat loss, this stands for
As Many Rounds As Possible, which
means you pick a bunch of exercises
and select a number of reps and
sthen try to complete as many rounds
as possible in a set period of time.
Your challenge is to decide whether
you're able to go flat out or whether
you should take it steady. After all,
you don't want to blow up half way
through.

EMOM: This one stands for Every
Minute On the Minute. So you pick
a move or moves, set your reps and
you complete them every minute. The
challenge here is to decide whether
you want to rattle through the reps
and give yourself time to rest or
whether you want to take is slower
and sacrifice your rest time.

Sample muscle building week

Here's what a typical hypertrophy week looks like

When we set out the fat loss example we just outlined one session. For muscle-building, it makes more sense to set out an entire week because that shows you how each body part fits into the micro-cycle. There are a number of different ways that you can create a muscle-building split and we go through the key ones in this section. In the week-long example on the following pages we've outlined a push/pull split. That means that sessions alternate between being made up exclusively of either pushing exercises or pulling exercises. We've done this because pulling or pushing exercises tend to work well together. For example, if you do a bench press, which is a pushing move, that will work well with a triceps press-down, for example, because you'll have begun to work your triceps in the bench before fully exhausting them in the press-down. The push/pull also works well because it gives you four work days and three rest days, which gives you plenty of recovery time while allowing you to complete a useful amount of work.

SEVEN-DAY SPLITS
When people are creating their programmes they usually think in terms of weeks. So they fit all of their workouts into a seven-day period. This is the easiest and most convenient way of arranging things but it isn't the only way. You could, for example, use a nine-day micro-cycle if that's the best way to ensure that you target each muscle group sufficiently. But for beginners, we'd suggest starting with a seven-day split.

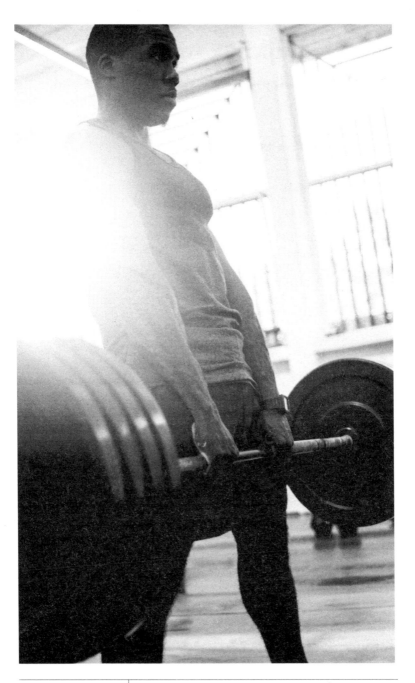

Muscle-building workouts

Here's how a full push/pull week split might look

Monday - Push 1: **Upper body**

Exercise name	Sets	Reps	Rest
1. Barbell bench press	4	8	90 sec
2. Cable chest flye	3	10	60 sec
3. Barbell overhead press	4	8	90 sec
4. Dumbbell lateral raise	3	12	60 sec
5a. Cable triceps press-down	3	15	60 sec
5b. Cable triceps overhead extn	3	15	60 sec

Wednesday - Pull 1: **Lower body**

Exercise name	Sets	Reps	Rest
1. Kettlebell swing	3	10	60 sec
2. Barbell deadlift	4	8	90 sec
3. Single-leg Romanian deadlift	3	10	60 sec
4. Barbell good morning	3	10	60 sec
5. Machine hamstring curl	3	15	60 sec

Friday - Pull 2: **Upper body**

Exercise name	Sets	Reps	Rest
1. Lat pulldown	4	8	90 sec
2. Seated cable row	4	8	90 sec
3a. Dumbbell prone row	3	10	60 sec
3b. Dumbbell prone reverse flye	3	10	60 sec
4a. Inline dumbbell biceps curl	3	12	60 sec
4b. Seated hammer curl	3	12	60 sec

Saturday - Push 2: **Lower body**

Exercise name	Sets	Reps	Rest
1. Kettlebell goblet squat	3	10	60 sec
2. Barbell back squat	5	5	120 sec
3. Leg press	3	10	60 sec
4. Dumbbell lunge	3	12	60 sec
5. Calf raise	3	12	60 sec

Training splits

The key splits that you can use to structure sessions

WHOLE-BODY SPLIT
What is it? This split involves sessions that work your entire body, so you may do one move each session that targets a particular muscle group, such as your chest or back.
Benefits: It's beginner friendly, because you're not asking each muscle group to complete a large volume of work within each session. It's also suited to those who are more interested in fat loss than building muscle.

Drawbacks: Because you only have time to do one move per muscle group, you won't properly fatigue your muscle fibres, which means you're not maximising your muscle-growth potential. It's only really an option for complete beginners or those who can only train once or twice a week. Once you get past the beginner stage, you'd be better off with a different split, if building muscle is your main goal.

UPPER/LOWER SPLIT
What is it? Each session is made up entirely of either upper body exercises, such as bent-over rows, bench presses and shoulder presses, or lower body exercises, such as squats and lunges. It works well if you can train four days a week, because you'll do two upper body and two lower body sessions.
Benefits: This is a pretty flexible and accessible way to train. It also ensures, if you're training four times a week,

that you train your legs twice a week, which is two times more than a lot of guys! It can also let you target a body part twice in one week, which is likely to give you a better outcome than only training the body part once a week.
Drawbacks: This is a perfectly good way to train. If you're quite advanced, there's an argument to say that the sessions will be too general and won't give you enough time to properly fatigue a target muscle group.

ANTAGONISTIC SPLIT

What is it? This is where you train two 'antagonistic' muscle groups per workout. Antagonistic muscle groups are ones on opposing sides of your body, such as your biceps and triceps, your chest and back and your quads and hamstrings.

Benefits: This is a good way of maximising the intensity of your session while also properly fatiguing each muscle group. For example, if you use antagonistic supersets you may do a chest move followed by a back move so while you work one muscle group, the other recovers. You can easily do three supersets per workout, which will let you properly fatigue the target body parts.

Drawbacks: There aren't many but the big one is that you'll probably only train each muscle group once per week, even if you're training four times a week.

BODY PART SPLIT

What is it? You dedicate each workout to a single body part, such as your chest.

Benefits: You will absolutely annihilate the target body part during the session. Doing five or six moves that focus on the same body part in one session is a tough but effective way of ensuring that you squeeze every ounce of capacity out of your muscle fibres. It's not where we'd suggest you start if you're a beginner, however.

Drawbacks: You're pretty much guaranteed to work each muscle group only once per week, which may not be the best way to progress. It's also possible that you're just not up to devoting a whole session to a single body part, and that your time could be used more effectively by introducing a second body part into the session. You'll also probably need to train about six times a week.

Anatomy of the perfect rep

Use this advice to get more out of every rep

Is there such a thing as the perfect rep? Maybe, maybe not. Regardless, your aim every time you pick up a weight should be to chase perfection because the closer you get to that, the more you'll get out of your session. Here's what you can do to optimise your approach.

Understand the technique: Before you even start your rep you should have a thorough understanding of the correct technique of the lift you're about to perform. You should also understand which muscles the exercise will work so that you can focus on them during the lift.

Use visualisation: This is something that elite athletes use all the time and there is evidence to show that visualisation techniques can improve performance outcomes. So before you start your set, mentally envisage yourself executing the perfect rep. Think about the movement pattern and visualise yourself lifting with strength, intensity and control.

Breathe right: This is an easily overlooked component of a rep. Correct breathing technique can act as a cue to your body as well as encouraging your core to engage. Before you lift, take a deep breath and contract your abs. Hold the breath as you perform the eccentric (lowering) phase of the lift and exhale during the eccentric (lifting) phase. Don't hold your breath for multiple reps because this will raise your blood pressure.

Initiate with the target muscle: It's so easy to get the rep off to a bad start by letting an unintended muscle in on the lifting action. Take the lat raise. A lot of people initiate the movement by shrugging up their traps when they should really be aiming to isolate the delts. Do be aware o the muscle you're trying to engage and be disciplined with how you move. It can take a while to be able to do this but it's a skill you need to practise.

Mind-muscle connection: This is an old school bodybuilding idea but it turns out that the big guys were on to something because recent research has suggested that thinking about the target muscle during a set can improve your results.

Perform a peak contraction: This is essential if you want to maximise the outcome of every rep. Take the biceps curl, for example. When you raise the weight, at the top you need to squeeze the biceps hard. This part of the contraction will ensure that your muscle fibres are working at their maximum capacity.

Keep the eccentric slow: This is relevant if you're aiming to build muscle. It's less important if strength if your primary focus. The eccentric is the lowering phase of the lift, such as lowering the bar to your chest during a bench press. To maximise your hypertrophy gains you want to use a roughly four-second eccentric. You don't have to use the same speed of lift all the time - its just a guide and a reinforcement of the idea that you shouldn't rush your reps because it's time under tension rather than the number of reps you perform that will have the biggest impact on your results.

Contract the agonist: This isn't essential for all moves but it can be really useful for certain exercises such as the biceps curl. The agonist muscle is the one on the other side of your body to the one you're working. So if you're training your biceps, the agonist if your triceps. To put this into action, when you lower the weight in a biceps curl, squeeze your triceps momentarily before starting the next rep.

Make every rep look the same: The point here is that you want your technique to be consistent. You will undoubtedly find the tenth and final rep of a set much harder than you found the first. And if you're using the right weight then you should only just be able to complete that tenth rep. Even so, it should look pretty much the same as the first. Sure, your face may contort a bit because you're working at maximum capacity but you shouldn't sacrifice technique in order to complete the rep.

Make some noise: A good indication that you're working hard enough is that you need to make a few grunts to help you complete the rep. This doesn't mean that you should make gratuitous noises but if you never need to make a sound, we'd question wether you're putting in sufficient effort.

Advanced protocols

Use these tactics to take your training to the next level

 Supersets: A superset is simply two exercises performed back-to-back with little or no rest. You could do a set of barbell bench press and go straight into a set of bent-over rows. There are a couple of reasons why you might want to utilise supersets. The reduced rest periods make them a time-efficient way to train. The reduced rest periods also increase the intensity and the fat burning effect of your sessions because while one muscle group recovers, another one is working. You can also use supersets to increase the demand on a target muscle by performing agonist supersets, which is where you pair moves that work the same muscle group, such as an incline dumbbell curl and a preacher curl - both of which target the biceps. Doing two moves that target the same muscle group is an excellent way of maximising muscle fibre fatigue but isn't a beginner-friendly way to train.

 Tri-sets: This is where you perform three exercises back-to-back without rest. It's an advanced training protocol, so it isn't one for beginners, particularly if all three moves target the same muscle group. You can use it as a way of working a target muscle from different angles. If we take the biceps, you could train three different positions of flexion by doing an incline biceps curl, a standing hammer curl and an EZ bar preacher curl. In each instance, the range of motion and the wrist position is different, so you're challenging your biceps in a range of ways in a very short space of time.

 Giant sets: This involves four or more exercises done back-to-back and is really only for advanced lifters. It's also probably only useful for smaller muscle groups, such as your biceps. If you tried to do it for your legs you'd get so tired so quickly that you'd have to use a low percentage of your one-repetition maximum, which means you wouldn't be working in a very effective hypertrophy range. That's not to say you wouldn't experience a hypertrophy effect, or that the protocol can never be used in that way. It's just something to be mindful of.

Drop sets: This is a tough but effective way of taking your training to the next level. Drop sets, in their simplest form, involve completing a number of reps to failure or near failure with a certain weight. That weight is then immediately reduced (by how much depends on your experience, your recovery speed and your goals), before you perform more reps, again to either failure or near failure. From there you can either finish the set or you can do another 'drop'. How many drops you do depends on your goals and experience but usually one or two will suffice. It's a really tough way to train so we'd only advise using it on one or two exercises per workout.

Pyramids: A pyramid involves increasing your rep count each set before reducing them again. So, for example, you may do 6 reps in set 1, 8 in set 2, 10 in set 3, 8 in set 4 and 6 in set 5. The theory behind it is that it probably takes you a bit of time to warm up when you lift so you'll often find that you're strongest on your second or third work set. But after that you may start to fatigue, so as your capacity to lift reduces, so do the reps.

Rest-pause: This is similar to drop sets in some ways, but instead of reducing the weight at the end of the set when you reach technical failure, you take a brief pause of, say, 15-30 seconds before lifting again for as many reps as possible. You can then do another pause before lifting again. How long you rest and how many reps you perform will depend on your experience, your goals and your speed of recovery. Interestingly, people recover at significantly different rates, so if you and a training partner both perform the same number of reps with the same weight before resting, one of you may be able to do twice as many reps as the other after the pause.

Create your own plan

Here's how to arrange the key training variables

Training split: There is no perfect split but there are splits that are more suited to people at different stages of their training journey. We'd only ever recommend whole body splits to beginners or those who are only concerned with fat loss, for example. You don't have to change your training split all the time but we'd generally advise against only ever following one type of training split. The best one for you is also the one that you enjoy the most, that you feel able to attack and the one that gets the best results.

Exercise selection: This is one of the most important elements of any plan. One of the big questions is the ideal ratio of compound (multi-joint) and isolation (single-joint) exercises that you should include. Traditionally, those prioritising strength might have a bias towards compound moves and those prioritising muscle gain would have a bias towards isolation work but that's not a hard and fast rule. We'd advise you to focus on the tried-and-tested exercises that give you the biggest bang for your muscle-building and strength training buck, which are the exercises we've outlined in the previous chapter.

Number of exercises: There's no perfect number of exercises per session but a rough number to aim for is about six. The number will depend on how many sets you're doing and what percentage of your one rep max you're lifting. You also want your session length to be about an hour, so doing 20 exercises in a two hour session is unlikely to be an optimal approach.

Exercise order: We'd suggest putting big compound moves at the start of your session so you can do them when you're fresh to lift as much weight as possible. Generally, the more technically challenging an exercise, the earlier it should be in the workout. Your isolation work should generally be at the end of your workout, unless it's the second move of an agonist superset, for example. And abs moves should be the final thing that you do. You may, however, use a light-ish exercise before your main move to excite your central nervous system and increase your potential in the big lift. Doing a few light kettlebell swings before a heavy deadlift session, for example, is a good way of getting your system fired up and ready to lift.

TAKEAWAY TIP: You don't have
to constantly reinvent your
workouts. Small adjustments
can also give you big benefits.

Sets and reps: This is something that you'll tweak endlessly. The classic
starting point for sets and reps is to perform 3 sets of 10 reps. That's great,
and will take you quite far, but you do need to look beyond that if you want
to maximise your gains. Generally, as sets increase, reps go down, and
vice-versa. So you might do 5 sets of 5 reps for a big compound move like
the squat. You'd also tend to do lower reps for the big moves. There's little
value in doing heavy doubles for biceps curls, for example. But there is
value in doing sets of 15 or 20 for your arms to make sure you fully fatigue
your muscle fibres.

Rest: The rest you take should roughly correspond with the reps that you
perform. Generally speaking the fewer reps you do, the longer your rest
should be. That may sound counterintuitive but because you lift a higher
percentage of your one-repetition maximum when you do low reps, it takes
your body longer to recover from the exertion. You may take 90-120 seconds
rest when dong 5 sets of 5 reps but only 60 seconds when doing sets of 10 or
12 reps. Typically your rest between exercises might be slightly longer than
your rest between sets.

Tempo: This is the speed at which you lift and is the most overlooked of the
training variables. There are four phases of each rep in which you can adjust
the speed, and they're as follows:
Eccentric phase - when you're lowering the weight.
First pause - this occurs at the bottom of the move (such as the bar on your
pecs during the bench press).
Concentric phase - when you're lifting the weight.
Second pause - this occurs at the top of the move (such as just before your
arms reach lockout during the bench press).
Tempo is expressed as a four-digit number with each digit representing the
time in seconds of that phase of the lift. So a 4011 tempo for a bench press
would be a four second lowering of the bar, no pause, a one-second push
back to the start and a one-second pause before starting the next rep. The
total length of the rep is called the 'time under tension'. For hypertrophy,
aim for a total time under tension each set of about 40-70 seconds.

How to keep a training diary

Record your efforts to track your progress

Keeping a workout journal is one of the easiest but most effective things you can do to ensure that you stick to a training plan and make the progress you want. All you need to do is record what you do in the gym. This will help you stick to the plan because if you don't have a record of what you've lifted then it's almost impossible to really know if you're making progress. If you have a written record of what you have lifted you can use it to make sensible incremental increases in the weight you lift next time you attempt that exercise. Our advice is to get a notebook or a dedicated workout journal, take it on to the gym floor and fill it out between sets. If you've never done this before, ensure that you fill out the basic workout details as an absolute minimum and, if you can, try to include other items of information as outlined below.

WORKOUT DATA

You should record the number of sets and reps you perform for each exercise. Also note down the tempo of the lift as well as the rest you take between sets and exercises. The other important item of information is the weight you lift for each set. Having this information is the most basic way of assessing your progress.

NUTRITION INFO

It is useful to make a note of what you eat before, during and after your sessions so that you can assess how your nutrition intake is affecting your performance. Write down what you had for your pre-workout meal and when you had it, as well as any pre-workout supplements that you've consumed. If you take on anything during a workout, even if it is just water, note that down too. The final element to record is what you eat for your post-workout meal.

EXTRA ANALYSIS

If you are new to training you may find that recording tons of information every time you train is overwhelming. If that's the case, stick to the basics. But if you can deal with it, more information will help you better analyse your performance. Write down the time of the workout and how much sleep you got the night before, and rate your quality of sleep out of ten. After each session, note what went well, what could be improved and anything that you'll try to do differently next time to boost your performance.

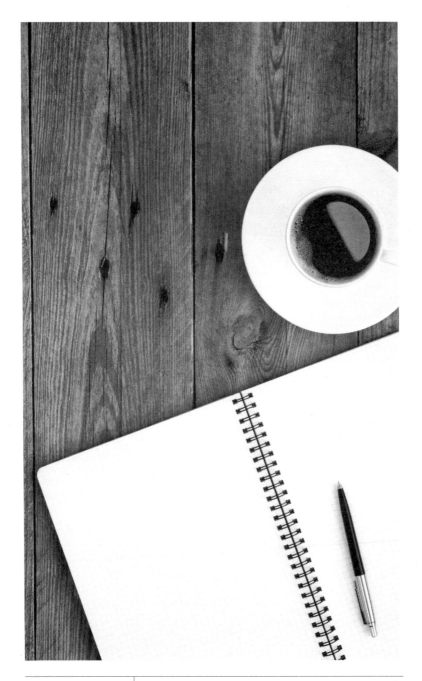

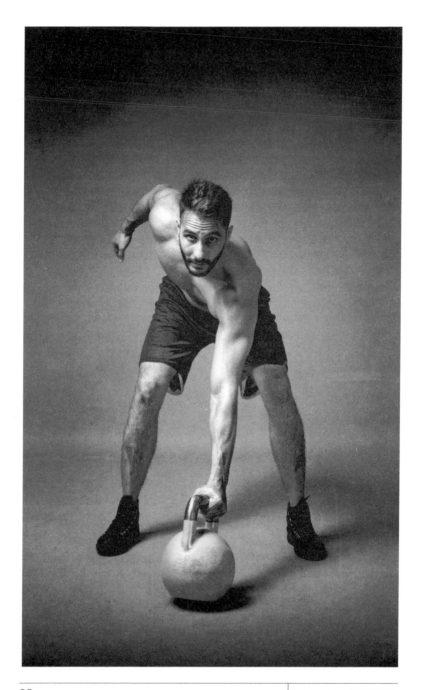

The key to training success

Here's what really matters when you step into a gym

 Consistency counts: Perhaps the biggest single factor in your overall progress is consistency. Without it, it is incredibly hard to make real and lasting progress. Let's say you do an outstanding session but then you do nothing for the rest of the week. That won't work. Neither will putting a few good weeks together before taking a few weeks off. But if you train consistently and you use the information in this book then you will make progress.

 Application of tension: This is almost always overlooked by inexperienced gym-goers and it is often ignored by more experienced exercisers too. In order to grow a muscle you need to properly apply tension to that muscle. That means minimising momentum and, instead, properly contracting the target muscle. Take a dumbbell biceps curl, for example. If your upper arm comes forwards during each rep that's a sign you're taking tension off the biceps. You should also take every opportunity to rinse everything out of every rep. If you squeeze the target muscle at the top of the rep, that will improve the quality of contraction.

 Focus on form: As an extension of the previous point, it's paramount that you lift with proper technique. Lifting with poor form will mean you miss out on potential gains at best and injure yourself at worst. Lifting with proper form can be tough psychologically, because it may force you to reduce the weight you're lifting, but in the long run it will be worth it.

 Make an effort: If you want to make serious training progress then you're going to have to train hard. It would be great if you got amazing rewards for half-effort sessions but it doesn't work like that. If you want to make progress you're going to have to work for it. You're going to have to go to places that make you feel uncomfortable and you're going to have to overcome the voices in your head telling you to stop. The good news is that if you do put the effort in then you will be rewarded.

Training glossary

Key workout terms explained

1RM Abbreviation of one-rep max, which is the maximum weight you can lift for one rep of an exercise with correct form.

Aerobic energy system The chemical and metabolic pathways within cells that need oxygen to create ATP. The aerobic energy system uses oxygen and fatty acids, as well as the products of glycolysis, to create ATP. Aerobic energy systems provide ATP at a much slower rate than anaerobic energy systems. Slow-twitch muscle fibres rely primarily on the aerobic energy system.

Agonist muscle The primary muscle involved in causing movement.

AMRAP Abbreviation of As Many Reps As Possible, which is a set where you do as many reps as you can with correct form, either in a set period of time or before reaching failure.

Anaerobic energy system The chemical and metabolic pathways within cells that don't need oxygen to create ATP. The recycling of stored ATP by creatine phosphate and glycolysis are both anaerobic energy systems. Fast-twitch muscle fibres rely primarily on the anaerobic energy system.

Antagonist muscle A muscle that can move a joint in the opposite way to the movement produced by the agonist.

ATP Abbrevation of adenosine triphosphate, an organic chemical responsible for transporting energy in all cellular processes in the body. It is required for muscular contraction, and the more ATP you have and the better you are at processing it, the stronger you are. It can be produced in three ways: the recycling of previously stored ATP by creatine phosphate; through non-oxygen dependent glycolysis (glucose metabolism); and through oxygen-dependent metabolism that utilise fatty acids (oxidisation).

Compound lift An exercise involving movement in two or more joints, such as the squat (hip, knee and ankle) and overhead press (shoulder and elbow).

Concentric contraction A concentric contraction of a muscle results in its shortening, which occurs during the "lifting" phase of a given exercise. When you curl a dumbbell up towards your body, that's a concentric contraction of your biceps muscles.

Creatine phosphate A molecule that helps recycle used ATP. When you have higher levels of creatine in the bloodstream, your muscle cells can produce ATP faster, helping you to train harder for longer.

DOMS Abbreviation of Delayed Onset Muscle Soreness, which is muscular aches and pains you feel after a hard workout. Also known as myositis.

Drop set A set strategy in which you perform an exercise to complete or near-failure, then reduce the weight and continue. You can do multiple 'drops' in a drop set.

Eccentric contraction An eccentric contraction is the lengthening of a muscle under load, which occurs during the 'negative' or 'lowering' phase. When you're lowering the bar to your chest during the bench press, there's an eccentric contraction of your chest muscles.

Exercise The lifts you perform in a given workout, which determines which muscles or muscle groups you train in that session.

Exercise order The order in which you perform the exercises in a workout, which helps determine the training stimulus on your muscles.

Extension An extension movement increases the angle at a joint between two parts of the body. Straightening your elbow in a cable rope triceps pressdown is an extension movement, as is standing back up from the bottom position of a squat, which uses hip and knee extension. Extension is the opposite movement pattern to flexion.

Failure The point when your muscles momentarily stop working and won't let you perform another rep.

Fast-twitch muscle fibres
Also known as Type IIA or Type IIB, these muscle fibres rely on glycolysis (the breakdown of glycogen) to create ATP to fuel muscle contractions. They get their name because glycolysis produces ATP much more quickly than the oxygen-dependent process used by slow-twitch fibres. Fast-twitch fibres are larger, can generate much more force, and have more potential for enlargement than slow-twitch fibres, but they fatigue much more quickly. They're used when lifting heavy weights or sprinting. Strength training increases the size and number of fast-twitch fibres, making muscles bigger and stronger.

Fatty acids Fatty acids are both important dietary sources of fuel and an important structural component of cells. They are used to create ATP, in the presence of oxygen, when muscle cells are using the aerobic energy system.

Flexion A flexion movement decreases the angle at a joint between two parts of the body. Bending the elbow towards you in a biceps curl is a flexion movement because the angle between your forearm and biceps (upper arm) decreases. Flexion is the opposite movement pattern to extension.

Frequency How often you train a specific muscle or muscle group in a given period, typically each week.

Glycogen Glucose stored in your muscles that is used during glycolosis to create ATP.

Glycolosis The metabolic pathway that converts glucose into ATP.

Hypertrophy Greek for "excess nourishment", hypertrophy is an increase in the volume of a muscle or organ caused by the enlargement of its cells.

Isolation lift A lift involving movement in only one joint, such as the biceps curl (elbow) and leg extension (knee).

Isometric contraction An isometric contraction is when a muscle contracts but without significant movement. Your abs and lower back muscles contract isometrically when you squat or overhead press to keep your torso stable during the move, but aren't involved in lifting the weight directly.

Lactate/lactic acid A by-product of glycolysis. It can be used by aerobic energy systems to produce more ATP through a process called the Krebs cycle.

Rep Abbreviation of repetition, a rep is the completion of a given exercise through its entire range of motion from the start (top) position to the end (bottom) position and back to the start.

Rest The time you spend recovering between the last rep of one set and the first rep of the next and the time between exercises.

Set The number of times you perform a certain number of reps.

Slow-twitch muscle fibres Also known as Type I fibres, these muscle fibres rely on oxygen and fatty acids to produce ATP to fuel muscle contractions. They are so-called because the oxygen-dependent process they use to produce

ATP takes much longer than the process that fast-twitch fibres use. Slow-twitch fibres are smaller and generate less force than fast-twitch fibres, and have less potential for enlargement. However, they are very resistant to fatigue and are used for everyday movements and endurance exercise.

Stabiliser muscle A muscle that contracts without significant movement to maintain posture or keep a joint in a fixed position.

Straight set With straight sets you do all the sets of the first exercise, labelled move 1, then move on to exercise 2, and follow this pattern until you've done all the sets of the final move of the session.

Stretch reflex When a muscle is lengthened under load during the eccentric phase a rebound effect takes place, similar to a stretching of a rubber band. This is why it is harder to start a bench press or squat rep from the bottom as opposed to the top because you must initiate the movement without the aid of the stretch reflex.

Supercompensation The period after training and recovery when you're fitter and stronger than before. Training in this window will result in further gains in strength, size and fitness. Training before this

window opens - not having enough recovery - can result in overtraining, while training after it has closed - leaving too long between workouts - limits your ability to make size, strength and fitness gains quickly.

Superset In a superset you do a set of the first exercise, called the A move, then do a set of the second exercise, called the B move.

Synergist muscle A muscle that assists the agonist muscle in a movement.

Target muscle The primary muscle being trained during an exercise.

Tempo The speed at which you perform each rep. It is detailed by a four-digit code that represents in seconds the time you take to lift and lower a weight, as well as pauses at the top and bottom.

Triset In a triset you do a set of the first exercise, called the A move, then do a set of the second exercise, the B move, then do a set of the third exercise, the C move.

Volume The amount of work you make a muscle group or groups do in a given session or over a certain time period, such as a week or a month. Volume is one of the key factors behind hypertrophy.